The Gift of Pain

The Gift of Pain

Transforming Hurt into Healing

Barbara Altemus

A PERIGEE BOOK

A Perigee Book
Published by The Berkley Publishing Group
A division of Penguin Group (USA) Inc.
375 Hudson Street
New York, New York 10014

Copyright © 2003 by Barbara Altemus
Text design by Julie Rogers
Cover design by Ben Gibson
Cover photo © by Y. Niwa/Panstock/Panoramic Images

First edition: September 2003

Visit our website at www.penguin.com

Library of Congress Cataloging-in-Publication Data
Altemus, Barbara.
The gift of pain : transforming hurt into healing / Barbara Altemus.—1st ed.
    p.   cm.
"A Perigee book."
Includes index.
ISBN 0-399-52778-8
1. Pain.   I. Title.
BF515.A58 2003
155.9—dc21   2002193074

PRINTED IN THE UNITED STATES OF AMERICA

10 9 8 7 6 5 4 3 2 1

For my precious daughter, Imani

An Elder's Words

In a dream, I listened as a wise man spoke
of the need for the people of the world to
transform their consciousness.
For he explained that we are living in the illusion
of being separate from one another, from all of natural creation,
and from our Creator.

He went on to share of
the pain that we carry within our hearts and souls
and how this pain serves to remind us
that we are out of alignment with the universal laws
placed here to guide us
and how we have forgotten
our true purposes in life.

Not understanding how to move through our pain
into joy
all too often we have inflicted more suffering upon ourselves,
our children, our mates, our communities, our nations
and the water, earth, air and other living beings,
pulling them into our own dance of demise.

He cried out softly, saying
listen with your hearts
for we are one global heart.
Become the beauty, peace, love and harmony
that you so long for in others.
Remember that it is in the silence of the mind,
the roaring of the wind,
the incessant rhythm of the waters
and the song of the birds
that we are reminded that
life is perfect.
You are perfect.

Move into your authentic selves.
Shine the radiance of pure love upon all those whom you meet
for there are infinite possibilities in this grand mystery
we call life.
Reach out for the calling.
Become the human being you have always been
and give your soul permission to soar.
For this life as it is given to us
is the most precious gift of all.

Move into the consciousness of caring for the sacred.

BARBARA ALTEMUS

Contents

Acknowledgments

Writing this book has given me the opportunity to heal and transform my life in ways that I could have never imagined. There are numerous remarkable people who have helped to make this book possible, and many others who through their presence and support have anchored me along the way.

First I want to thank my daughter, Imani, who inspires me endlessly with her refreshing wisdom, sense of humor, open and loving heart, spirited nature, and adventurous outlook on life. You were so enthusiastic about traveling with me and meeting the contributors in the book, and we shared the most amazing of times together. I thank you from the bottom of my heart for putting up with my endless hours of writing and editing—especially toward the completion of the book. When I became weary, I would peek in at you sleeping and be reminded that all is well, and that I am here doing what I am meant to do. In your own special way you always bring me back to my true self. Thank you for all of your love and support. You are the angel in my life.

I want to give a heartfelt thanks to my extraordinary brother, David. You have supported me in so many ways, but most of all by believing in me and lovingly standing by my side. Without your help, this book would have never been the same. You are the brother that every sister wishes for.

To my dear friend Miriam Lynette, thank you for consistently supporting me with your love, wisdom, and expertise. You are an editor extraordinaire, and this book sings louder and clearer than it ever could have without your help. It has been wonderful working with you.

Afrika, my sweet sister, thank you for sharing endlessly from the bottom of your heart your brilliant insights, your love, and your contagious enthusiasm. You never stopped believing in me and when my energy would waver, you always reminded me to shine my light.

Reverend Michael, my deep thanks for anchoring this book spiritually, believing in me, being a guiding light, and bringing special people into my life and into the book.

Thank you, Bernie Dohrmann, for sharing with me the spiritual inspiration you received for me to write this book. Without your clarity and heartfelt message, the book would have not come to be. I thank you for being the messenger of love that you are.

My dear friend Gay, thank you for loving me and insisting that we go to an IBI preview. If I had not gone, I would have never heard Bernie's message for me to write the book. I know you are smiling down upon us as this book comes to completion.

My beautiful sister Rose, thank you for always believing in me, sharing your loving spirit, and guiding me on this path.

To my literary agent, Roger Jellinek, you are a gift from the heavens. You have always stood by me, believed in me, and guided me in the direction I needed to go. My very deepest thanks for taking me by the hand and showing me the way to becoming a published author.

My dear friend Bob Gillespie, thank you for understanding from the inception of this book its true message and for supporting me in every way possible. Without your assistance the book would not be what it is today.

To my dear friend and coach Don Hallock, thank you for your invaluable guidance in discovering the deeper meaning of the gift of pain and for helping me to be able to express that in the book.

Thank you Michele, my beloved sister, for sharing with me your love and support. It has helped carry and sustain me.

Thank you Roy, for believing in me and the book, and for supporting Imani and myself in keeping ourselves healthy in mind, body, and spirit. Thank you Dr. Michael Masters and Drs. Kerry and Terry Haydel for keeping my body in alignment. And thank you Dr. Lou Jensen for your invaluable support in keeping my immune system strong through the long and sleepless nights working.

A heartfelt thank you to Jan, Justin, Jill, Tommy, Danielle, Joe, Kate, Will, Sonia, Hardy, Helen, Jeanette, Mia, Loreene, Gladys, Donald, Jimmy, Bridget, Jared, Noel, Topzyana, Duane, Milissa, Kristin, Helen T., Helen J., Irma, Beth, Liz, Alisha, Dawn, Paula, Wahopi, Elaine, Joanie Klar Bruce, Sue L., Lyla, Lehua, Eric, Nicole, Cynthia, and Mark, for believing in me. With your love and inspiration, I was constantly reminded that all things are possible.

Thank you to Beatriz Haymer for beautifully transcribing Rigoberta Menchú Tum's interview, and Debra Payne, Rebecca Smith, Sherry Stowell, Everlyn Aloya, Megan Metz, Dodi Gronau, Sharon Popp, Bevery Kaya, and Cristina Hernandez for your extraordinary work in transcribing the interviews. Thank you Dane Musik, for showing me how to use a computer.

Thank you David Altemus, Lisa Campbell, Sharon Popp, Justin Altemus, and Stewart Reiner for so generously sharing your office with me.

A heartfelt thank you to all of the contributors. In a most profound way you assisted me in my own healing and transformation and made this book possible. I know you will help countless others as well.

Thank you to Michelle Howry at Penguin, for doing such a fine job editing. It has been wonderful working with you. And thank you to Jennifer Repo, for believing in the book and contributing your editing expertise.

I want to especially acknowledge my mother and father, Sylvia and Jules Altemus, for without their guidance, love, and support from the other side, I would not have been able to carry out such an endeavor. Working alongside them has been a most awesome experience. Thanks Mom and Dad, for teaching me the true meaning of feeling connected.

And thank you Spirit, for without You, none of this would have been possible.

Introduction

As I disembarked the airplane, having traveled from Los Angeles to Honolulu, I took my young daughter into my arms and asked, from the deepest place in my soul, for the Creator to show me my life's work. I had just left my daughter's father and had moved to the Hawaiian Islands. Although in one way it seemed as though I had lost everything, I was also beginning anew with a multitude of possibilities and opportunities in my life. I had a willingness and openness to heal, and I felt I had been given the opportunity to heal and transform my pain.

Within two weeks, a dear friend of mine, the late Gay Baird, took me to a seminar that assists people in living and financing their dreams. I was inspired and interested in the projects people were discussing, yet I did not really know what I wanted to do with my life. I had been teaching for some fifteen years, yet I still felt boxed in, and as if there were more for me to do. After the preview I spoke to

Bernie Dohrmann, the founder of the seminar. He looked intently at me, in a very penetrating way, and said, "You are going to write a book about alternative ways of healing pain, and the book will lead to much, much more."

I immediately looked at my five-year-old daughter and knew that there was no way I could support her and write a book. I tried to block out his words, but they kept resonating deep within me. And over the next several years, I encountered extraordinary people who soon were to help finance my travels, support me in this project, and assist in connecting me to people I wanted to interview.

I had the opportunity to attend the IBI seminar in California on "working as a team to make our dreams come true." On the plane home, I experienced a tremendous inner journey. I heard a voice speak very clearly, guiding me that the book was to be about healers, visionaries, creative artists, and peacemakers who share their stories, life experiences, and perceptions about healing and transforming their pain. Ancient and alternative ways of healing were to be part of the book as well. The voice then mentioned numerous names of people to interview, including Deepak Chopra and Nelson Mandela, whom I had not met yet. I proceeded to call a Lakota (Sioux) medicine man to get his feedback, and he said, "Yes, write this book, and come back for ceremonies before you begin." I then called Dick Gregory, and he said, "Yes, write this book, this is one of your life assignments." Then Reverend Michael said, "Yes, write this book, but your life story needs to weave the entire book together."

The "much much more" that Bernie referred to prompted me to

invite Spirit to guide me. At the IBI seminar I experienced a vision of spiritual leaders from throughout the world meeting in a conference in South Africa. I saw this vision, like a movie in front of my eyes, as did another woman at the seminar. We became very excited that both of us saw the same vision. We were sharing our vision with Dr. Enrico Melson, who was the head doctor at Deepak Chopra's Center for Well Being, when one of the delegates at the seminar came up excitedly to share his own vision. He told us that he visualized HIV and cancer being eradicated with energetic medicine. Without wanting to interrupt him, I asked, "Was it in South Africa?" He was astounded and asked, "Yes, how did you know?" We all felt the synchronicity and the serendipity of our being brought together. This took place in 1994.

In 1999 another friend asked me how this book came to be written, and I recounted the vision of spiritual leaders traveling to South Africa for a conference. He said, "What you saw is what we're having in South Africa with The Parliament of the World's Religions. You must come and speak." I attended this conference in 1999 and brought Mayan spiritual leader Juana Vasquex de Arcon on behalf of Nobel Peace Prize Winner Rigoberta Menchú Tum, and served as her interpreter and translator. I felt that this was part of the unfolding of the vision I had had years before.

In 2002 I was to return to Africa as part of a Delegation to the World Peace and Prayer Day held in South Africa. Our delegation was led by Lakota spiritual leader Chief Arvol Looking Horse. Ela Gandhi, Mahatma Gandhi's granddaughter, hosted this ceremony on her grandfather's land in Durban, South Africa. It was a day when people of all faiths gathered on sacred sites around the world to pray for global peace.

On my personal healing journey, I have learned that everyone experiences pain—physical, emotional, mental, and spiritual pain. Pain is a wake-up call and it can trigger renewal, or entrenchment. Pain affects individuals, families, and nations, bringing forth their best and worst qualities. It can be felt as a sharp or chronic physical pain, or as a whisper in the night, a longing, a deep loneliness, an insecurity, an overpowering fear, or an excruciating assault on the soul. Many people go to extraordinary lengths to avoid pain, often sacrificing the quality of their lives to do so.

Some cultures help to buffer the effects of pain in people's lives with a powerful attunement to the cycles of life and their traumatic changes by using ceremonies that convey great importance and meaning, by reassuring family bonds, and by establishing beliefs that help to strengthen equanimity in the face of challenge. The standard Western methods of dealing with pain are to avoid it, deny it, medicate it, resolve it—make it go away. But pain can be used as a catalyst to help us transform our consciousness and live our lives in a more meaningful, fulfilled, and joyous manner.

Having a sense of connectedness is a powerful personal resource that can be cultivated. We are strengthened when we feel connected to our cultural and ancestral heritage, when we feel close to spiritual principles and our connection to a Higher Power, when we are aware of our connection to all people and living things, when we can understand the natural cycles of life, when we feel connected to the invisible world, and when we can be conscious of the unity and basic harmony of all of life. This is true strength and well-being.

Our beliefs that we live by are serving us well when we feel balanced, calm, joyful, loving, and close to people and to all of life. When we feel anxious, stressed, hurt, hateful, and separate, our belief system and our actions require change. Our beliefs greatly determine what we experience. Sometimes to lift ourselves out of pain, we must change our beliefs and what we tell ourselves about our experiences and expectations. We need to upgrade our truths.

We can create a life relationship that works better and better for us. We can discover and piece together a total context that promotes harmony and balance—a wisdom template. This is a book about the resilience of the soul, of human beings, of nature itself. We can see how resilient the people in this book are when faced with their pain and their challenges. They stand forth to show the way. All of us can continue trying and exploring, and we can help each other find the paths that work well. I invite you to share with me a most inspired journey of healing and renewal.

Chapter One

> *"I was a victim all of my life, and I was thirty-five years old before I realized there are no victims. It occurred to me, 'Then what does that make me? What am I going to be?' I was a victim of poverty, of abuse, of neglect, of incest. But I now know those experiences taught me what I needed to learn."*
> —Iyanla Vanzant

I found sanctuary huddled into a ball on the kitchen floor. Mom and Dad were fighting again. I was three years old and feeling frightened and alone. They continued to scream and yell until one of them noticed that I was eating a banana, the skin and all. Even at age three, I felt powerless over their arguments and felt as if I did not matter. In later years, to make myself feel more important, I lied to my friends in order to protect myself. I told them I had ten brothers and sisters, and even told some that I lived in a different house to keep them from coming close to my home and hearing the yelling and screaming that so often came through the kitchen window. At times I tried to holler over their fighting so the neighbors would think I was the problem. It seemed to me that the entire neighborhood could hear my parents, and often I felt sad and humiliated because people did know what was going on. They would ask me what the fights were about. Sadness and humiliation became a part of my growing up in my early years. It was a blessing that my sister was born when I was nine years old, because the fighting let up almost completely. This opened the way for me to have a most loving and devoted relationship with my mother and father.

I learned at an early age that one of the most important things in life is to strive for peace. When we have peace we are loving, affirming one another's worth, and making one another feel valued. In turn we feel joyful. When there is peace we feel rooted, connected to one another and to the values and principles of peace. Peace is a state of being and a state of consciousness.

On the other hand, when there is fighting, poor communication, or no communication within the family, this disconnection causes much pain and sorrow. Much family pain originates from feeling separate from one another and not knowing how to feel or get connected.

Much of my pain is rooted in my Jewish history. Some of my extended family perished in the Holocaust and others survived, scared and unable to heal their anguish. This legacy was passed down from my grandparents's generation, to my parents, and finally to mine. Not able to recognize nor express their feelings before the hurt turned into anger and rage, loving communication rarely found a means of expression. It was not in the good times that loving communication was difficult—rather, when we were hurting we did not understand how to affirm and support one another. This legacy of disconnectedness passed down in my family and millions of other families affected by genocide not only affects our family members but the perpetuators as well. All too often when we do not heal the abuse, we become perpetrators of more abuse, contributing to the endless cycle of pain.

It was precisely the hurt and pain I felt as a child that was a catalyst for my seeking spiritual roots and a better understanding of how to heal and transform my own pain. I was determined to break the pattern of emotional outbursts in my family and the violence I witnessed in the world. This propelled me to become a peace advocate and to learn about Native American spirituality. I cherished the Native American way of honoring all of life and holding a sacred place for every living being in the circle of life. And in time, I also became a therapist working with families in crisis. I believe that my personal quest for self-balance and harmony has led me to a much greater purpose of helping to bring about peace in the world.

In healing the pain I felt as a child I interviewed several amazing people who each inspired and guided me in my process of self-discovery and renewal. Their writings and personal stories have deeply touched my soul and given me the insight, strength, and determination to understand that when we have a pure and clear intention all things are possible.

We each have had common themes running through our lives. We have felt powerless, separate, abandoned, unsafe, and restless at various times in our family lives. But importantly, these experiences served as a catalyst, catapulting each of us onto a journey where we would discover how to become empowered and connected. We learned how to cultivate a sense of belonging and, ultimately, a feeling of safety and inner peace. We each continue on this journey today open to the multitude of possibilities for creating an even richer life.

Isabel Allende's writing is filled with deep reflection and spiritual resonance that soothes the soul and reawakens the spirit. In her work, I often see myself, the part of me that longs to be deeply authentic, renewed, and totally vulnerable in life. Isabel was an exile from Chile, forced to leave her native homeland after the military coup in 1973, so we were indirectly connected. My work as an advocate for peace in Chile involved getting safe passage out of the country for her uncle's family, the slain President Salvador Allende. I felt very close to the situation there because I was in Chile in 1971 during the revolution and I grew to love, respect, admire, and feel total solidarity with the people of Chile.

Isabel is one of the most highly praised and widely read writers to come out of Latin America. She has written such bestsellers as *House of the Spirits, Daughter of Fortune,* and *Paula.* She shares from the depths of her soul. And the wisdom, courage, and strength she has found within herself gives each of us understanding and inspiration to know that we too have the resources within ourselves to heal and transform our pain, when we intend to do so.

One of her first painful experiences happened when she was just three years old. Her father left the family and never came back, and she says that it changed her life completely. She says after that, "My mother was always sick and I had a feeling of insecurity that every-thing was going to collapse any minute, that my life was like a house of cards." Coupled with these burdens, Isabel's grandmother died when Isabel was still a child. Her grandmother was extremely im-portant to her and losing her was devastating. She shares, "Some-thing died in my life that was very important, and when my grandmother died my grandfather mourned her terribly. He dressed in black, painted the furniture black, and flowers, desserts, and music were banned from the house. So I spent many years of my childhood in mourning, in a somber environment, where nothing was happy or easy. And life was about suffering. Life was about pain. Life was also about giving, charity, and about discipline. Everything was strict. There was no music, no joy, no feasting, no partying, no celebration of life. I remember my childhood as dark and unhappy."

She also admits that her greatest fear was that her mother would die. But when her mother remarried a diplomat, instead of feeling safe and comforted, Isabel really started to feel loss. They moved from one country to another, and as she says, "The feeling of loss, of being lost, was frequent. Because I couldn't speak the language of the country, I couldn't even take a bus and go anywhere. There was a sense of physical dependency that if anything happened to these two adults, I would be really lost. I mean in Lebanon, you are really lost!"

In time Isabel was able to value her travels. She says, "The fact that I had to move from so many places to so many places gave me flexibility, a sort of capacity to adapt, that many people have not de-veloped. And that has been useful in my life." She also gained an awareness that people in the world are basically the same. She says,

"No matter how different cultures may seem externally, people react to the same things in more or less the same ways. We all want the same things. We all want to be heard. We want to be touched. We want our children to be safe. We want to avoid fear and pain."

Perhaps one of the most important insights from Isabel is the way she views how she changes. "I have never changed out of joy. Joyful experiences have not forced me to change. What forces me to change is something stressful, something very painful most of the time. That is what forces me to go inside myself and see what I've got to deal with. What are my resources? And by bringing those resources out to the surface and using them I learn what my strengths are. I needed to go through all the changes, all the exiles, all the losses in order to know that I can adapt. That whatever happens I will be sooner or later OK. But in order to learn that I had to go through those stages, and pain is a great teacher. I'm not afraid of pain so much anymore as I was before, not even physical pain." Over the years Isabel has grown to understand that she is more resilient than she realized and that her resilience has allowed her to face her challenges with courage, fortitude, and clarity.

It took me a long time to face my own challenges with clear focus, and I grew to understand that sometimes another person can help us in ways we could not have imagined. Such was the case when I met Joan Borysenko, Ph.D., author and pioneer in the mind-body health movement. I first met Joan in 1997 at the Body and Soul conference in Boulder, Colorado, where she was a keynote speaker. I had read her book, *Fire in the Soul*, which had helped me to understand that much of my family pain could be an initiatory ritual rather than a life sentence. But I was still struggling with issues of abandonment and victimhood, and her strength and courage taught me that I could move from being a victim to having self-mastery in my life.

It turns out that we have much in common, from our family pain to our interests in Native American spirituality and other forms of spirituality. She had served as an outstanding example of working to heal her pain with Mind/Body/Spirit medicine, and I was inspired by her success in healing her life and in sharing with many others through her books, lectures, and workshops. Joan is the author of several best-selling books including *Minding the Body, Mending the Mind; A Woman's Book of Life;* and *A Woman's Journey to God.*

Like Isabel, Joan's first sense of disconnection was when she was in grade school, because she never felt like she fit in. And that feeling persisted until she was in college. "I always felt that somehow I was on a different wavelength, that I had different values, different interests, and I felt generally disconnected from my peer group. Although I had very loving parents, I felt somehow rootless in terms of family connection. We had lots of grandparents and cousins around, yet I felt almost like a stranger around them."

Joan's mother emphasized that Joan should not be too smart, because "smartness alienates people," and ultimately she wanted Joan to marry a rich Jewish man who would take care of her. As Joan says, "I didn't share those values in the least. I was much more interested in spiritual and intellectual things. I really didn't care much about material things. Her constant harping on how I looked and what I wore, and wanting me to conform was incredibly painful because I just wanted to be myself. I can actually recall coming to blows with her for the first and only time in my childhood, at about sixteen, when I tried to leave the house wearing sneakers. And that was so unladylike as far as she was concerned, that she thought this was going to be the ruination of my future and that no nice boy would love a girl who left her house in sneakers. And that was really hard because there was no one to support me. She wanted me to live out her dreams, and I didn't want to do that."

Joan's father was a very vulnerable person. He was depressed. He had a nervous breakdown when she was about ten, after being held up in a store at gunpoint. Joan spent a lot of her time trying to make him feel good, and taking care of him emotionally. "He was also sweet, funny, and much more intellectually interesting than my mother was. But a disappointed person. My father forsook his dream to be a mathematician to go into his family business. His professor told him Jews do not get ahead in academia and he wouldn't make enough to ever get married. He went into the family business and then the liquor business. And was a disappointed man all of his life. And I ended up kind of holding a lot of the pain in that."

Joan lost her father at an early age. Joan's father died when he got cancer and was given a drug that made him manic. As a result, he jumped out of a window and committed suicide. This was incredibly painful for Joan because she felt that she hadn't kept him safe. She was a cancer researcher and worked at Tufts Medical School and had a grant from the National Cancer Institute and "all the information that I knew about cancer did not translate into anything that would help my father as a person or us as a family. It was hard. And then my mother suffered from survivor guilt, and I went into behavioral medicine to deal with the problems. I changed fields because of this pain. It was a turning point in my life." Joan decided that helping others would help her work through her own grief and loss. "I learned that I could not possibly stay locked up in a laboratory. That part of my own healing was going to have to be helping other people in similar circumstances."

So Joan left Tufts Medical School and joined the mind-body division of Behavioral Medicine at Beth Israel Hospital. They did clinical research trials that incorporated managing stress, mindfulness meditation, and yoga, and she has found this path to be a much more fulfilling use of her talents and gifts. Joan sees pain as something that, when you work through it, becomes a source of your strength. "I feel very complete with my relationships with both my father and mother. They each gave me gifts, including the gifts that grew out of the pain from both of them. I feel very complete with that." Joan came around full circle, from struggling with wanting to be true to herself in her teens to discovering, through life's challenges what it means to be her authentic self.

Like Joan, Iyanla Vanzant learned through turbulent and challenging times to find her authentic voice. Iyanla is the best-selling author of numerous books, including *In the Meantime* and *Acts of Faith*. And she is an inspirational speaker throughout the world. Iyanla has overcome much pain in her life that, sadly, began at an early age. She says, "My uncle raped me and I told my aunt and he denied it to my aunt. Nothing was ever said about it again. So that silence taught me not to speak out, not to speak out against injustice. And it also taught me that I didn't matter." Iyanla took that belief into her intimate relationships, resulting in a marriage where her husband cheated on her and beat her up. She constantly chose painful situations that mirrored how she felt about herself.

What changed her forever was when she heard God speaking to her. "I became really conscious the first time I actually heard God speak to me. I had gotten glimpses of it before but never like this time. I was lying on the grass under the sun, and I felt myself in the midst of this fog and I started breathing it and then I realized that I couldn't move and I couldn't open my eyes but I could see. I heard the voice say to me, 'What do you want?' And now I'm in my human body freaking out that I can't move. I realized this was God speaking to me, and why would God be speaking to *me?* And the voice said, 'God is speaking to you, what do you want?' And I panicked and I said, 'a car.' And the minute it came out of my mouth I said, 'Oh, F***!' I said the word, then I really panicked because now I had cursed in front of God. That's it.

"I was just freaking out on the grass, and the voice very calmly said, 'What do you believe about a car?' And I said, 'I believe you have to have money to have a car.' And the voice said, 'No, all you have to do is have an idea. If you have an idea of what you want and you believe that you can have it, you'll have it.' The fog lifted and of course I got up to haul my behind away from there 'cause I just knew I had lost my mind.

"I was on the ground of the convent of the Divine Mother. I ran around the corner, and there was this fourteen-foot statue of Mary.

She was facing this way so I went over there, and when I looked up, I fell onto my knees and I prayed. I think that was my first conscious contact, understanding, communication with this uniting force of God."

Her conversation with God changed her life, Iyanla says. "I don't know if everybody can have one of those experiences, but I would really recommend it, because you get real clear. I didn't need a preacher. I didn't need a priest. I didn't have to be a virgin. I didn't need to be wearing size 5. I didn't have to be blonde or blue-eyed. I didn't have to have teeth in my mouth. I didn't have to have anything but an open heart."

By that time, Iyanla had already been initiated into the Yoruba priesthood and had gone through workshops, seminars, and initiations, but she says it wasn't until God spoke to her that her life changed. Prayer is so important to her because she believes it keeps people connected to their Higher Power. She says, "When you pray, just talk, just open your mouth and talk to God, 'cause God is right with you. It's unfortunate that religion and irresponsible theology have made us think that there has to be a certain way and form to pray. That's very irresponsible of people to make us think that we're not worthy to pray to God. That causes pain."

Often when someone has had a painful upbringing, the sense of being a victim can follow them right into adulthood. Iyanla says, "If you think you deserve to be in pain because you have been told all of your life that something is wrong with you, that you are not doing it right, that you are not good enough, then you begin to believe that. You think that you are supposed to suffer and then you create your suffering. But today, twenty-three years later, I can say that I caused my own pain. In some cases I did not understand this. In other situations I understood and I resisted anyway."

Iyanla came to realize that our holding a belief in separation is fostered by our conditioning and programming. She elaborates, "This is particularly so for women experiencing who we are, what we are, what we are doing, what we can do, and what we cannot do. You take this to a deeper level when you talk about women of color in this society, because we are so conditioned as to what we can and cannot do. It is challenging, and to resist the challenge is painful—but it is more painful to not push beyond the barriers, to not challenge the stereotypes, and to not use our gifts, talents, and abilities."

Falling into the trap of feeling like a victim is widespread. Iyanla shares, "If you look at what a victim is, victims have to be hurt. I was a victim all of my life, and I was thirty-five years old before I realized there are no victims. It occurred to me, 'Then what does that make me? What am I going to be?' It took a while of flailing around in self-flagellation to figure out what I'm going to be. I thought I was a victim of poverty, of abuse, of neglect, of incest. But I now know those experiences taught me what I needed to learn."

Iyanla believes that the pain we feel inside is often caused by a sense of separation. She says, "There is only one cure, and that is remembering that we are always connected to God and each other all of the time. I think that is the ultimate healing lesson, and it is not necessary to create a big ritual about getting back our connection. We don't have to have a ritual to plug into God. The minute we decide to do it, it will happen. And although the principles of faith, trust, belief, and intent may sometimes be hard for us because we cannot always see the reasons and benefits of these things, the more we embody these qualities, the more we move from pain into joy."

Iyanla says, "You can refer to God as Universal Intelligence, The Divinity within me, Universal Mother, Holy Spirit, Great Spirit, Creator, whatever, because God will meet you where you are. If you are into rocks and crystals, God will meet you there. If you are into angels, God will meet you there. If you are into Jesus, Buddha, Krishna, Allah . . . God will meet you where you are! And we need to understand that and stop trying to do it right. And wherever we are, to whomever, call out . . . help me, I am in trouble, could you give a sister some help?"

Today, Iyanla makes us all laugh and cry and feel from the depths of our souls with her wisdom and messages through her books and TV appearances. She has inspired me with her clarity, loving heart, and persistence to keep following her dreams. Her intention of not wanting to hurt kept her open to the possibilities of healing her pain. She is a great inspiration, reminding us that when we are willing to heal, all things are possible.

Jack Canfield encountered similar lessons about healing pain in his past. As best-selling coauthor of the popular *Chicken Soup for the Soul*® series, self-esteem expert, and motivational speaker, he has guided me and countless others with his determination and forthright approach to living out his dreams.

Healing his past has taken Jack down many different roads. When he was fifty-six years old, Jack was in therapy and a repressed memory emerged. He remembers, "Here I am fifty-six years old and it was only a month or two ago in my therapy that I dealt with a memory that I had repressed, that my father put a 45-gun to my head one day, and said something to the effect of—I was about six years old at the time—'If you don't calm down and be quiet, I'm going to shoot you.' And that terrified me. I think that's one of the reasons I've been a big proponent of the gun control movement and a pacifist. I think that's part of my essential nature, but I also think that it's part of a psychological wound that makes me want to not have that happen to other people. I would say that I'm probably ninety-five percent healed from that, but there are little things that still emerge from my pre-six-year-old time of life." Jack's mother divorced his father when Jack was young, and he was certainly affected by those early years. He knows that he wasn't deeply nurtured or supported by his parents and that for a long time trusting people was very difficult for him.

Jack talks about the turning point in his life, when he began the process of looking honestly within himself and examining his feelings. It all began around 1967. There was a part of himself that was so hungry for that kind of emotionally deep connection that he took a lot of weekend personal growth workshops. "I would even volunteer to be on staff for these workshops so I could get in for free. Then I moved to Amherst, Massachusetts, and started a retreat center for these kinds of workshops, and I also started doing ongoing weekly therapy. I began to go much deeper in dealing with the pain of my childhood—my sense of abandonment by my mother and my fear of my father. But it was a gradual process that took place over time."

Jack's biological father left when Jack was six and Jack never saw him again. However, a year ago Jack was able to get into contact with his half-brother and half-sister. He says, "We've had some nice conversations. Although we haven't met yet personally, we met on the phone numerous times. And sometime this year I'm going to go to Chicago and spend time with them. They told me that when our father remarried their mother, he joined Alcoholics Anonymous, and he was just a totally delightful guy. I think it had been the alcohol that was running him before. So it's sad that I didn't get to know him better."

Jack knew that the only way to move through the pain of violence was to seek help learning how to turn within, and in so doing, discover his own resources to heal. As he became clearer and stronger he began to share with others what he had learned. And sometimes, giving back to others is the most healing action we can do. When we heal and transform our childhood pain, we are given the opportunity to discover new meaning and purpose for our life. The hurt can serve as a gift, helping us to clarify what we want in life, and how we can best share that with others. The transformation occurs when we are seeking to grow and we begin to recognize that life is filled with infinite possibilities. We are each given the ability to make choices and to learn and to grow from our choices. On this journey, we can learn to take responsibility for our own lives rather than blame another for our pain. And perhaps we can even understand that those who have been abusive to us in our lives have helped us to discover qualities within ourselves such as compassion, strength, generosity, and honesty.

Gerry Jampolsky, M.D., psychiatrist and founder of the Center for Attitudinal Healing, and best-selling author of *Love Is Letting Go of Fear, Teach Only Love,* and *Good-bye to Guilt,* has contributed so much to the healing of children and people around the world because of his own journey to heal himself.

As a child, Gerry did poorly in school and did not understand why. He was dyslexic and flunked kindergarten. He felt a sense of separation from his peers, and thought he was a disappointment to his parents and his teachers. He says, "The love I received was conditional. If I got good grades then I would get more love. Besides being dyslexic, I was kind of a hyperkinetic kid who tended to spill his milk and do all other kinds of rowdy stuff, so I had an extremely poor self-image growing up. Most of it was not a happy time."

Gerry now understands that he walked around feeling like a victim. He got into the University of California, Berkeley with a D-minus average and remembers a professor once telling him to never try to write a book. Of course, Gerry did write very inspiring books and has helped thousands of people with his work. But he didn't have any kind of transformational process until he was fifty years old and was introduced to *A Course in Miracles.* At that time he was an alcoholic and in the middle of a very painful divorce. He says, "I heard an inner voice saying, 'Physician heal thyself, this is your way home.'" He also believes that our pain is much deeper than we think. He says, "Suffering has psychological components, often there is guilt, there are grievances and also there are unforgiving thoughts. It's important to really take a look at our grievances and then release them. We need to forgive ourselves and forgive others."

Gerry's life is testimony to the fact that we should always listen to and trust our inner voice. His teacher told him he should never try to write, but he listened to his inner guidance and penned extraordinary books. Gerry became the outstanding teacher and therapist he is today not in spite of his life experiences, but because of them.

When someone sets out to heal the past, their journey will be unique because what one person needs will be different from another. And what one finds will be different, too. Joan Borysenko found that being part of the early mind/body health movement was essential to coming to terms with her father's death. Mindfulness and hatha yoga became a way for her to stay in the moment and not run from her feelings. Iyanla, on the other hand, found a direct connection to God and understood that she could no longer live with blaming others for what happened in her childhood. And Jack Canfield and Gerry Jampolsky's willingness to continually heal themselves allows them to help others.

In my own determination to not repeat my parents' turbulent past, I've faced challenges and overcome obstacles that I never thought possible. A lot of pain is caused by living and obsessing about our past or worrying and fretting about what will become of our lives in the future. But I have learned that feeling abandoned by my parents when they were fighting was driving me to make choices and to form beliefs that were not always healthy. I was not loving and caring to myself.

Most of us consider our origins to be our families. That may only be true in a worldly sense. Certainly our families have an immense amount to do with the shaping of our lives. We can consider our family as a starting point, but what we will find is that we have other origins, such as our origin in the Spirit. And knowing this is a good start to healing oneself.

Chapter Two

Redefining Success and Failure

"As a person begins to become conscious of what they really are and what their unlimited potential is, they start to live more from a 'vision space' than from a 'pain space.' "
—*Reverend Michael Beckwith D. D.*

I sat in my classroom disillusioned, angry, and hurt. I was in a Ph.D. program at the University of California at Irvine entitled Comparative Cultures. The program was recognized for its progressive curriculum focusing on issues of alienation and oppression within cultures. But ironically, I was feeling more and more isolated from my instructors and classmates as my studies continued—we studied so much theory that there was little, if any, time to share what was in our hearts and minds. I also began to find it more difficult to talk with the people closest to me, because my academic studies were teaching me to theorize and intellectualize to the point of creating distance between us. The connection that I once had with my loved ones was suffering greatly. In my classes I kept asking, "Does anyone here want to talk about how we can become better human beings?" A few students in the program felt as I did, but by and large, we were the minority. I felt estranged in this doctoral program and not at all enlightened by the higher learning experience.

About a year into the program, Native American leader Ernie Peters told me about the Longest Walk, a spiritual walk across the country led by Native American spiritual leaders and undertaken by people from across the world. The Walk began on February 12, 1978, in California with a couple of hundred people and was completed in Washington, D.C., six months later with more than 35,000 people. One of the main purposes of the Walk was to protest ten congressional bills designed to take away Native Americans' rights and an eleventh bill that would take away freedom of speech for all North Americans. Ernie told me that the Longest Walk in a spiritual sense would take back the land, as was foretold in Native American prophecies, from the West to the East. He said, "Barbara, on the Longest Walk you will learn what it means to be a good human being." My soul just opened up, and my heart knew that I had to be on the Walk.

This brought a great deal of challenge and excitement to my life— leaving the doctoral program and spending the next six months walking, living in tents, and being among people from almost all of the Native American nations as well as people from the four corners of Mother Earth. According to the mind-set at the time, it was un- thinkable to leave such a successful Ph.D. program in order to join a grassroots walk across the country. But my mother's full support of my participation gave me the strength, determination, and will that carried me forth in each step I made across the country and still today lives within my heart—carrying me higher and higher with each life endeavor I accomplish.

On the Walk, it became clear that my former notions of success and failure were no longer serving me. I had often measured success by prestige and status, and I had thought that these guidelines would sustain me and carry me through life. But the Walk made me realize that being tied to this belief system caused me much pain and distress, and ultimately that it was holding me back from living a full life. I decided to redefine for myself the meaning of success and failure, and in doing so, live my life in alignment with values and principles that resonate in my heart and soul. I began to see that success and failure can be measured in how well we are able to convert our pain into a larger purpose.

One such person who has reevaluated success and found new meaning is world-renowned actress Goldie Hawn. People who are in the public eye, such as actors and musicians, often struggle with issues of success and failure. Fame and fortune give one the appearance of having achieved ultimate success, and therefore happiness. But, as Goldie revealed to me, material success can actually be a challenge to overcome and on the way to knowing one's higher self.

Goldie discovered at a young age that, although her success in Hollywood made her appear to "have it all," deep within herself she felt uncertainty and fear. She shared with me, "When I became successful I was filled with confusion as to who I really was. I felt like I was free-falling. Everything that I related to as normal was being challenged, and my reality shifted so drastically—from having nothing to having what people thought was everything. I experienced a deep anxiety. I lost my sense of self and was unsure of who I was.

"I left home when I was nineteen. I studied dance, and it became my vocation. I traveled around the country, happily dancing for a living. I never gave it a thought that I would be plucked into the elite world of luminaries, not to mention that I would become one! I was young and never had to question my identity. When strangers started to take photographs and want autographs, it felt so foreign. Everyone seemed to know me, but they didn't . . . and my reaction to all this frightened me. I went through emotional symptoms that were uncharacteristic. I stayed in the comfort of my apartment, drank tea, could hardly eat. I suppose one could call it an acute nervous reaction.

"Anxiety-ridden, I sought professional help. That was the turning point and the beginning of my life. The veil slowly lifted, illuminating a greater understanding of the nature of the mind, my mind." This allowed Goldie to start trusting in her inner life as a haven rather than a fearful place.

Today, Goldie believes that it's important to honor the difficulty in our lives, as well as the successes, and she teaches her children to know what their dreams are and to own them. She says to them, "Conduct your life accordingly. The most important thing is the process, the process of life, the stepping stones that we take. Joyfulness is in the details. And don't miss those, because that is what really forms you as a human being. And don't focus only on what you believe is going to make you win."

When her children ask Goldie for advice, she tells them to "hold on to your dream, but don't be attached to it. Live your enthusiasm and stay curious. Your ideas will change, and movement is the life force. Embrace change. I pray your passions are not always self-serving. Give back, enliven the spirit, enlighten, be a messenger of joy. Live in the moment!"

For Goldie, meditation is very important to keep a sense of balance in her life. She says, "I know that when I do my meditation I ground myself back into the real truth, which is that none of us, basically, are in control of things. We are instruments. And when I bring the light through my body it's very powerful and I have a great sense of well-being. We cannot expect someone else to do it for us. We cannot wait for the light to enter by itself. We have to be willing and ready, and we have to put this into motion ourselves. Meditation is very important for that. It leads to a respect for all of life as well as devotion, gratitude, and wonder. It also helps us to take ourselves out of the equation and become a witness. If we are able to become a witness to everything, including ourselves, then we are dealing from our Higher Self, which transcends ego."

Through the more challenging and painful times in life, Goldie has learned the meaning of compassion and of having gratitude. She is also continually redefining what "success" means to her, and how she can use her success to affect others' lives. She is an advocate in support of Tibetan and Native American rights and spirituality, as well as a goodwill ambassador for peace. She shares, "Looking at this beautiful life I have now, I feel that it is my duty to give back. I have received an unbelievable amount of light and love, and just this incredible sense of fulfillment. I think we're in a global crisis right now. I do what I can do to be able to give back to the world, to shed light, to bring awareness, to be effective. To help make a shift."

Like Goldie Hawn, Reverend Michael Beckwith has encountered his own struggles with defining success, and today he offers others a way to higher truth. Reverend Michael Beckwith is founder and spiritual leader of Agape International Center, a transdenominational spiritual community based in Culver City, California. Dr. Beckwith has worked with His Holiness the Dalai Lama and numerous spiritual leaders in an effort to create world peace. Along with Arun Gandhi, he is a national co-director of A Season for Nonviolence, which teaches and practices the nonviolent principles of Martin Luther King and Mahatma Gandhi.

Like so many young people, Reverend Michael, in his teens, became cynical and disillusioned about life. In an effort to heal his personal pain he became politically active, and his thoughts were revolutionary. "I believed that the system we are living in was corrupt and did not lend itself to people's freedom, creativity, and expression. Rather it was a materialistic system driven by economics and not necessarily about human qualities and thoughts about humanity."

Reverend Michael began working with an organization that was about creating change, only to become more disillusioned because, as he says, "I remember looking at the people in the room during a meeting and thinking, 'If we were to take over the world, would the world be any better?' I looked around the room and saw power struggles going on. There was jealousy and a lot of ego in that group. I realized the world probably would not be any different if they were in charge of it. The problem was not just about revolutionizing a system and making things better, even though there probably are better systems. It was something deeper than that, but I did not know what it was."

Confused and dismayed, he redirected his energies and began pursuing a different type of success. He went back to college and made some money hustling on the streets. "My dream was to go to medical school and then give my services as a doctor. But at the same time I wanted to be financially secure. I blocked most of the pain of not knowing what and who I was by keeping busy with a lot of external activity and drugs. I thought I was having some kind of psychotic break or going crazy because I was leaving my body a lot, hearing messages, seeing things, and having a lot of prophetic insights, visions, and dreams. At the same time I was living in this very materialistic world and trying to make a lot of money. It was a very confusing and painful time in my life."

A turning point was when he started to have a recurring dream that continued for almost a year. "At the culmination of the dream, two men held me down and I was stabbed in the heart; I let out this bloodcurdling scream and then I died. When I awoke my perception was different. I saw things in a new way. I reconnected with my original intention for being here on the planet and with the part of myself that wanted to be of service and to create. I saw something that I would now call Life or God—it was everywhere and it was in every-thing."

It was at that point that Reverend Michael began to understand that all the crises in his life at the time served as a birth into a greater avenue of awareness. "It was as if one week I was operating from one place and the next week I was delving into a new place called God. To the outside observer it looked as if I had just flipped out. But they did not have the privilege of seeing the internal process that had been going on for over a year—the visions and the dreams and the death in the dream."

For Reverend Michael the dream was a dream of transformation. He interpreted it as, "The self who had sold out to materialism was killed off. I was transformed inside, and my real self came to the sur-face. The personality that had been molded by society fell away and a tender, new being emerged. I could see and experience it happen-ing. I became both the observer and the observed. I saw the knife go-ing into my heart and I actually felt the pain as if somebody were plunging a knife into my heart."

Interestingly enough, Reverend Michael for a number of years *had* heart pains, usually at times of great change and transformation in his life. He explains, "I would have to slow down my breathing and take shallow breaths because it was excruciating just to breathe. This became an indication to me that I was expanding and at the same time trying to hold on to the past.

"When I first began to have these severe pains, I went to medical doctors and had chest X-rays and cardiovascular examinations. There was nothing wrong—it was totally on the level of my spirit and psyche. I think that is a metaphor for everything."

From this experience Reverend Michael learned about the pain or suffering that comes from resistance. He often refers to the pain as being "the effort it takes to cling to an old thought pattern, and the effort it takes to not change and to stagnate."

Reverend Michael grew to understand "that as human beings we are all at a particular level of spiritual evolution where we have to consciously participate in our own growth. There is an abundance of resources to support us in the process. To the degree that we are not consciously participating in becoming conscious, God shows up as the face of crisis and pain, to assist us on our way. The only thing we are left with after a crisis is our existential awareness of the presence of God or our real values."

To aid him in his own growth he studied ancient texts from some of the Eastern religions and philosophies such as the *Bhagavad Gita* and the *Vedas*, as well as the writings of great masters including Sri Avrobindo and Paramahansa Yogananda. He also studied a lot of New Thought teachers, such as Joel Goldsmith. And, primarily, he practiced stillness, mindfulness, devotional prayer, and, vipassana meditation. All these texts encourage becoming awake. For Reverend Beckwith this means a connection with God. He says, "At first I felt a growing surrender to the presence of God, which has now become a complete surrender through a dedicated practice of meditation and study. This has become my way of life."

For myself, the Longest Walk became integral to my own awakening. I started learning about other people, spirituality, and connecting with the natural creation in ways that can only be experienced firsthand. Many myths were dispelled and truths illuminated. The lessons learned moved my soul and have been everlasting. I discovered the importance of becoming rooted to life principles and practices that feel true to my heart. In creating roots I gained an understanding that all begins from within. My life started to feel more joyous and peaceful the more I connected with nature and people who were like-minded. Although I joined the Walk politically minded, by the time we reached Washington, D.C., I was embracing the spiritual and creating my own definition of success. My quest became one of understanding my own spiritual roots, having the opportunity to be tested day after day, walking, enduring on all levels, and assisting myself and others in cleansing what was not necessary in our minds, hearts, and bodies. It was indeed a spiritual journey.

I was able to complete the Walk and, in a way, complete a type of spiritual commitment. I had a deep sense of fulfillment and success because of my new altered perceptions. But when one isn't able to accomplish a particular goal, especially of a spiritual nature, there is an emptiness and a deep sense of failure. John Funmaker, spiritual advisor and drug and alcohol counselor at the Robert Sundance Family Wellness Center in Los Angeles, knows what it's like to struggle with these issues. When John was nine years old, one of his uncles told him about going on a Vision Quest, a four-day fasting ceremony done alone in the wilderness. John explains, "He took me up on the hill and I stayed there for two days. I planned to go back before the end of the summer to complete two more days. I was not able to, for some reason. And I always remembered that I still had to go back up on the hill."

It wasn't until years later that another Native American spiritual leader offered him the chance to do the ceremony again. "We made all the preparations, and I made a commitment with the Sacred Pipe. I fasted for four days, four nights, no food or water, and I went through a really difficult time. I did a lot of thinking, and a lot of praying, meditating, a lot of crying, and I was trying to come to some understanding, trying to come to some place where I would not be so self-destructive. I wanted to live, and I wanted to be happy. So I think that that was really a good ceremony, it gave me time to think and time to focus on myself, and look at myself. That was a major turning point in my life when I went through that ceremony."

John's completion of his Vision Quest changed his values and brought greater depth and new direction to his life. I understand this well, because when I had finished the Longest Walk, I certainly had a deeper sense of who I was, and more importantly, what values I wanted to honor. Suddenly the Ph.D. program didn't seem that important to me. But, sometimes, to find our true calling in life, we must make difficult choices and painful sacrifices that may seem like failures. Blase Bonpane found that following his true calling in life would indeed mean facing obstacles that would alter his life and force him to stand up for what he truly believed in.

Blase Bonpane is an ex–Maryknoll priest who has dedicated his life to helping create peace in war-ridden places of the world such as Guatemala, Iraq, Colombia, and Chiapas, Mexico. He founded the

Office of the Americas in Los Angeles to educate people about what is happening to people in Central and South America. Standing up for what we believe in can be extremely liberating, but it can also cause us much pain. Blase knows this all too well from working as a Maryknoll priest in Guatemala during 1962–1965, a time when the United States was involved in Vietnam, and in the post–Vatican II period. At that time the priests were given the right to use their own judgment when working with the hopes, desires, and anxieties of the people. It was a politically dangerous time, and the efforts of the Maryknoll priests to aid the poor were seen as subversive. Blase remembers, "We were surprised because the biblical literature itself is biased on behalf of the poor. We were then pursued, our students were sought after, our center was bombed, our place was machine-gunned, and I was thrown out of the country." This was an extremely distressing and painful time for Blase, since he had grown to love the people, culture, and the land of Guatemala, and he felt the calling to help make a difference in these people's lives.

But sometimes we are presented with situations that show us clearly who we are and what we are here to do. After Blase left Guatemala and reported back to the Maryknoll headquarters in New York about the appalling treatment he'd endured there, the leadership's response caused him to question what he was doing for the order. He says, "At the time our superior general was very much in sync with U.S. policy and with U.S. agencies—FBI, CIA, it was part and parcel of the whole fabric. And so he gave me a gag order. Told me not to write, not to speak, not to organize, and to go to Hawaii immediately, which I did. I woke up the next morning in Honolulu and asked everybody—was I really not supposed to speak, write, or organize, and forget Latin America? And they said, 'Absolutely, these are the conditions of your being here.'"

This was a major turning point in Blase's life. He knew he had to live by his conscience and stand by his truth. It was clear that no authority, government, or person was going to tell him who he was or how he was going to live his life. More than ever he felt the calling to follow his Spirit.

Blase went to the *Washington Post* and told his story identifying the Green Berets operating in Guatemala and the napalming of villages. The piece was written and printed, titled, "Guatemala, Our Latin Vietnam." Blase knew he had contradicted orders, but he decided to sacrifice his own career in order to make a difference for the people of Guatemala. He spoke his truth and shared what he witnessed firsthand. And the world listened. He started speaking around the country and worked with the peace movement that opposed Vietnam. By this time, he had separated from the Maryknoll society, which was a difficult move for him. He remembers, "I can't imagine a pain greater than the pain of leaving my clerical career, at that time. It was very, very hard because I had been an extremely 'successful' priest. I had been a regional superior of the area, I enjoyed responsibility, I enjoyed my work enormously, I also I felt that that was my calling. And then I began to realize there is a distinction between vocation and career. I learned that my vocation is to do what I have to do today, no matter what the demand is. My career is what I happen to do for a living. Your vocation may interfere with your career, but your career is less of a thing than your calling. I really sensed in those years that my vocation was to follow the Spirit, even if it took me right out of this very 'comfortable' situation in the clergy. I had to follow that Spirit right out of the practice of the priesthood as an institutional priest, and that was very painful but very excellent in the response."

Blase was given the opportunity to face the deepest truth of who he is. "I had to look at my role as a priest and realize that I have to be something deeper than that and to give up that role, though technically you never give it up. I mean if we're going by Catholic theology, you're always a priest. I'm still a priest, but I had to reject that particular authority that was directing me to do things that were outside of my inner calling."

Perhaps Blase best describes what he has learned in these words: "It sounds contradictory to say 'happy are we who mourn.' The point being that facing head-on the mourning of the world, including our own mourning, and trying to deal with that mourning, we are able to transform our pain and the pain of others. 'Happy are you the peacemakers, you shall be called the children of God.' It's important that we face the pain of conflict and we ask how we can transform that pain. This is what healing is about."

It isn't always easy to stand up for what we believe in and to live our truth. When we remain strong and rooted in spiritual principles and feel connected to our source, we are nourished and sustained. Blase wonderfully inspires us to listen carefully to what our life's calling is, and in so doing, be divinely guided in carrying out our life's work. We discover that when faced with painful and difficult challenges, we will be given the tools and the qualities that will assist us in our healing and transformation. And by being true to ourselves, we can perhaps encourage others to do the same.

I have one particular memory of the Longest Walk that will forever shape the way I understand life, because it gave me the faith and belief in infinite possibilities. A tornado was about to hit the town we were in, and the news services advised everyone to find shelter. At the time there were nearly a thousand people on the Walk. So the spiritual elders had us join together in a circle for prayer. The sky was threatening, with huge black clouds looming overhead. I had never seen anything like it in my life. According to the radio broadcasts, the tornado was destroying people's homes and moving over seventy-five miles per hour. As the tornado headed closer, suddenly the winds became calm and as we looked overhead, the sun began to peek through the darkened clouds and an eagle majestically circled overhead, reminding us that we were indeed blessed, protected, and loved. This experience reawakened our awareness of the possibilities of prayer, connecting us once again. We felt our oneness with one another and Mother Nature and our Creator.

It is part of the human condition to feel doubt and disconnectedness at various times in our lives. When we're overcome by these feelings it's often necessary to just still our mind, and let the thoughts move through. Rigoberta Menchú Tum knows about the importance of everything having its appropriate time. She is a celebrated Guatemalan Indian leader and Nobel Peace Prize winner, and the author of two best-selling books—*I, Rigoberta Menchú* and *Crossing*

Borders. Rigoberta was forced to flee from Guatemala, deeply traumatized by the violence inflicted on her community—including the murders of her brother, father, and mother. She has since shared with the world her people's sorrow and today heads the Rigoberta Menchú Tum Foundation, based in Mexico City, Mexico. When faced with her own doubts she says, "When I feel that the struggle I am making is useless, when I feel it is a failure, that it isn't giving results, it is wearing me away, in those moments I feel I don't recognize human beings as a part of my species, I see them as strangers. I must take a time of silence to reflect, to think. Usually, I go back to nature. I go back to my parents' property, the place I struggled so very much, to reclaim again. It is the place where my parents' house was, where there is a total silence, a cloud forest. And I think. I think about the world and return to that place. Or, I simply think of nothing. I just observe the clouds. I observe the sky, the land, the smallest mountain animals. I observe the darkness. I attempt to observe the stars and the world, to breathe the air and give myself time. I'm sure with eight days of being in a moment of reflection with nature, I will want to start over again. After this I am full of much energy to begin again, after some time of reflection. I feel very capable to take on whatever type of tasks for whatever time is necessary."

Because of the nature of her work, Rigoberta often faces moments where her mission for peace seems insurmountable. She faced one particularly challenging obstacle while writing her book—Rigoberta could not read. It is an arduous task to write a book, but an even more challenging endeavor when one has never read a book. Rigoberta shares, "My first book, *I, Rigoberta Menchú*, the story of my life, was recorded in twenty-six or twenty-seven hours and was written with various friends. At the time the book was written, the world outside of Guatemala, outside of my village, Chimel, was unknown to me. I was rapidly learning many things, but what I knew was insufficient. So I didn't even have a clue of the importance of a book. In all my life up to that time I had never read a book. I never thought of reading a book. Even now, reading books is one of the skills I have acquired, but have not fully developed. I read only the parts of a work that interest me, the parts that I connect with or that are about a concept I am trying to grasp. The desire I had to write that book was so I could be heard, and they heard me. This was a major turning point in my healing."

For many years Rigoberta could not read her own book. She says, "I could not read the book, first of all, because of the pain it caused me and secondly, because we Maya are very mystical about time. If there is a work that I've done, that work becomes a mystical part of my life and that work is sacred. It is a magical work. It is full of life, and hope, and denunciation, and anger, and violence. So I always considered the book as my ambassador, to shatter the silence. The book, *I, Rigoberta Menchú*, became one of the first big goals I have achieved."

Rigoberta explains that in all periods of history, the perpetrators write about their victims. She says, "They write using their own approach and destroying the dignity of their victims. Many historians reveal that the perpetrators not only torture their victims, they torture their victims' history. This is why I feel proud to be one of the writers who tells about the dignity of the victims. I have struggled for the truth of the victims, for the truth of the indigenous communities, for the dignity of our youth, our Maya children, for indigenous people from all parts of the world, for the dignity of ancient cultures. I still struggle against the genocide."

After being awarded the Nobel Peace Prize in 1992 for campaigning for human rights, Rigoberta's mission didn't stop. She says, "Receiving the Nobel Prize is like having a platform and a big microphone. It helps me with my mission. It is a mission of struggle and of work, of sacrifice, of effort. It is an example of a woman like me, who was born into picking cotton and coffee, who was born into misery, poverty, and neglect, who was born abandoned far away in a place without a name. I was a servant and cleaned bathrooms and mopped floors. I did many jobs that dignify women and dignify people. I should claim the Nobel Prize as a platform to claim dignity and justice for all. I think it is something very great, very sacred. I feel this Nobel Prize is active. It is proactive and so I struggle. I have no limit for working with the Nobel Prize. I believe it is a blessing from the gods because I did not receive it because of my own merits. I received it because our *nahuales* are at my side, they accompany me, they love me, and have in some way punished me in order to put me before these things that sometimes are extremely challenging."

On her own healing journey, Rigoberta has not forgotten the multitudes of people who have suffered or are suffering. Her goal is to be a guiding light for them. Rooted in Mayan culture and spirituality, she was taught values and life principles that have helped sustain and nourish her through her pain and in her healing and growth. Rigoberta explains, "We Maya believe the more positive energy we have in the depths of our hearts, at the bottom of our work, in the spirit of our work, the better the intentions carried by any of our actions, be they spiritual, political, or practical, the better will be our energy and the more difficult it will be to overcome that good energy. There is no negative energy that can destroy it completely. So, I practice this."

Today Rigoberta attributes many things to helping her transform her hurt into healing. She says, "I could sit for a long time digging in the dirt. One day. Two days. I don't have a limit for being with the land. Being with the land changes my life. It changes me completely. I also know how to pay my tributes to all the *nahuales* when it is necessary or when I think of it, not when I have problems, but when I have successes as well.

"On the Mayan calendar there is a time called Toc. It is a time when we must all pay our gratitude for the bad and the good. We—my husband, my son, and I—always do this." And in her healing she also believes there are bad things for which we must be profoundly grateful, because as she says, "In the end, that evil has become something good for us, a blessing, or it has become something positive in our lives. It may affect us at the moment, but afterward the positive energies begin to yield advantages."

In her healing, Rigoberta has learned about the importance of us each meditating a moment on ourselves. She says, "I meditate on myself. And I ask what have I done? Is what I have done good, or have I not done good? Are there negative things in my own attitudes? We have the ability to meditate and reflect upon an attitude, to say, 'No, that was not good.' And to say, 'That was bad; that should not happen.' The ability to meditate and reflect, to realize the negative, is a great human quality that all human beings possess."

Rigoberta exemplifies what it means to grow into our infinite possibilities. She is fully connected to her ancestral ways and grounded in principles of global peace even though she has experienced the most horrific genocide upon her family and her people. She comprehends what it means to be connected, rooted, one with herself and all of natural creation. Her inspiration is carried by the winds across borders, ethnicities, genders, languages, and economics. She illustrates to millions of us how to live our lives more fully. Rigoberta truly understands the beauty of transforming her pain into some meaningfulness.

Like Rigoberta Menchú Tum, Dick Gregory has known all too well the pain of inequality and injustice. He, too, has become an eloquent and impassioned spokesperson for peace and justice.

Dick is a renowned author, public speaker, brilliant comedian, leading civil and human right's activist, and a man totally committed to non-violent social change. He uses fasting, prayer, and other non-violent means to stir people's consciousness and move their hearts. I first met Dick on the Longest Walk. His profound understanding of truth and justice was expressed in a most heartfelt manner and moved me deeply.

Feeling ashamed of who we are and looking outside of ourselves for an identity is hurtful and all too prevalent in today's world. Dick's way of relieving the pain he felt as a child growing up poor and treated unequally as an African American was to go to the movies to watch his hero John Wayne on the screen. "I felt so ashamed walking home from the movies so I would start to walk like John Wayne, spit out of my mouth like a cowboy, and get the feeling that I was someone important and powerful."

That feeling was something Dick constantly sought, unaware of his dependence on other people's approval. He shares, "I became the greatest athlete in the history of Missouri. And that feeling was a great feeling. Almost like the movies. And then I became a great entertainer. That surpassed being an athlete. And then I went into the Civil Rights Movement and I saw all them white folks surroundin' the airport waitin' for me to land, and that's when I truly became John Wayne. And I loved it."

Dick began to understand that there was something greater than being a Hollywood celebrity, when he was "just being in the movement and seeing the evilness and seeing decent people not get scared and I'm scared. I'm sitting there and I'm looking at them folks stand there, lookin' at them women, all women. Corns on their feet, bunions, standin' there, waitin' to die, if that's what it comes to. And I just sat there and I thought to myself, 'You know these people never get their name in the paper.' And I just know right then, I'm on the side of right, don't need to be validated by the *New York Times, Washington Post,* or NBC or CBS. It was a wonderful feeling.

"The movement opened me up to where I could accept certain things. And I looked around and I took my time and began to understand the true meaning of love, of peace, that you don't have to have whiskey and sex to have a party. And then I realized it's a quiet thing within me."

Dick decided to learn how to fast, as a further form of protest against Civil Rights violations. He went to Dr. Fullerton, one of the world's greatest authorities on fasting. "She told me exactly what was going to happen to my body on the first day, the second day, the third day. And it happened. That's what saved me. The UPI was there, the AP was there takin' pictures every day. They were seeing the weight loss and publicizing it every day. I was enjoying that, but that was showbiz, you know? Nobody had ever done it in America, when the world was lookin' at it. And I loved, God I just loved it. When you fast, you're really on nature's operatin' table. I mean, I didn't realize for a long time that a real fast is not even drinking water. The word *fast* means to abstain from. It was a long time before I got into real spiritual fasting, where I just prayed. I went to Canada and checked into a house, just rented a house all by myself and fasted and prayed for forty days."

Dick is a great teacher for so many of us who have looked outside of ourselves for validation and meaning. He was considered by the press and television to be a celebrity, but it was in his work in the Civil Rights movement, alongside elderly women, and in his quiet moments of contemplation, prayer, and fasting, that he began to honor and love himself and His Creator. He grew to understand about the sacredness of life. From a loving and empowered place, Dick continues to motivate and inspire people throughout the world to walk in truth and to stand up for justice.

Similar to Dick, Martin Sheen has grown to understand that there are two distinct realities in life—one outside of ourselves and one from within. Martin reminds us that it is up to each one of us to choose which reality we are going to be ruled by.

Martin Sheen is a world-renowned screen actor, star of numerous motion pictures, including *Apocalypse Now,* and a Golden Globe Award winner for best actor in the hit TV series *The West Wing.* He is also widely recognized for his political activism around environmental issues and human rights.

During the filming of *Apocalypse Now,* Martin suffered a heart attack. This painful event served as a wake-up call and a catalyst to help him look honestly within himself and question how he was living. From this experience, Martin began to transform his life. He shares, "I think that the most important lesson I learned was that I chose the situation which caused the heart attack. I placed myself there and I was willing to accept the responsibility for it, and that was in large measure the most healing aspect of the journey. I also learned if you can imagine yourself healed, you can become healed. And you'll find the means to reach that level of freedom and imagination.

"My recovery was very much guided by my teacher—who happens to be my wife, Janet. She was by my side within hours after my heart attack. She ran down the corridor beside me as I was being pushed on the gurney and whispered into my ear, 'It's only a movie babe. You take it too seriously. It's only a movie babe, that's all it is.' And that was the beginning of my recovery."

Martin's healing helped him to recognize that "all of us are co-creators, and the most important element in our healing is ourselves. And from that, other realizations seem to come." Martin knows that pain is an important element in our growth, in our reality, in our humanity and of our journey. As we experience personal pain, we can see it in others and we can relate to them. We can help heal our own pain best by helping to heal the pain of others. And in this way, all of us become wounded healers.

All too often we become stuck in our pain. Martin has learned that "pain is only part of life. It is not the purpose of life and it is not the end of life and it is not life itself. It's part of the journey to freedom. I think our purpose here is to win our freedom, consciously. You can't do it through drugs or alcohol, you can't do it through sex, you can't do it through political power, you can't do it through money or clothes, and you can't do it through the color of your skin. It must be done through your consciousness. Your acceptance of who you are, where you are, and what you are. And you're let out on your own and you can choose from then on."

Martin doesn't experience the reality of any given day without experiencing some measure of pain, regret, guilt, doubt, fear, and anxiety. He says, "These are all very painful emotions. I think what motivates me is the reality of the pain of others. I'm able to see myself in the kinds of pain that I'm not always able to articulate, yet I've seen in others. Very often it's unspoken first, it's in body language, sometimes it's things people don't do not only the things that they do do. So I try to gauge my pain barometer by the pain I witness in others. And the reverse is true as well. The joy barometer is equally as powerful. Tears come to my eyes with equal ease to measure the pain and the joy. You can't have pain without joy and you can't have joy without pain. Both are fleeting and they are equally important."

Giving is an integral part of healing for Martin. "The giving of yourself, or your vulnerability, the showing of your love—no matter how much pain you're in, there are others in more pain. If you're able to get outside yourself a little bit, you'll see someone in worse shape. I think we are all greatly healed in the surrender to others. It's hard to do because we're so egocentric, but I think that is the most complete healing and the longest lasting, basically seeing ourselves in others. And we realize we don't have it so bad and we're never alone, and the universe is a friendly place."

How extraordinary that Martin was able to place more importance on the inspiration and teachings he received from within himself, rather than from the star-glittered world of Hollywood and its promises of success and happiness. Martin exemplifies how we each can take a seemingly tragic and painful event in our life and discover the gift lying just beneath the surface. The gift can be the answer to show us a better way to live our lives and to fulfill our dreams.

Like the others in this chapter, Chief Arvol Looking Horse has chosen to follow his heart. Although at times this has caused him much pain and heartache, it is precisely what has given him the strength to become who he is today. Chief Arvol Looking Horse is the Spiritual Leader and Keeper of the Sacred White Buffalo Calf Pipe of the Lakota, Dakota, and Nakota, otherwise known as the Great Sioux Nation. He has been an ambassador for peace in Iraq and elsewhere, and has shared his wisdom at the United Nations and with other spiritual leaders across the globe. He is carrying forth the Lakota, Dakota, and Nakota prophecies of peace and unity with the International World Peace and Prayer Day.

Arvol was chosen to be the spiritual leader of the Great Sioux Nation at a young age, and the expectations were sometimes overwhelming to him as a young boy. "At the age of twelve, I became the nineteenth generation Keeper of the Sacred C'anupa Calf Pipe, the Sacred Pipe. I was so proud that I was given this headdress, and was honored as a young man in that way. Then shortly after, I experienced a kind of cultural shock. Suddenly there was a lot of anger, hatred, and jealousy. I got caught up in all the things that were not good. I was hurt every which way possible, spiritually, mentally, physically, and emotionally, because it felt like there was no place for people like me, a spiritual leader. Where was I to fit in as a Lakota man?"

Government boarding school was an especially painful place for Arvol. "People openly cut down Indian people and kids called each other 'Chief' like it was a bad thing. When I was growing up the majority of people were Christianized and there was little respect for the traditional Lakota ways. This hurt me very much and caused me much anguish and sorrow."

Arvol remembers, "At school, my teacher told us we would never be leaders in the world. He said we could only become carpenters, auto mechanics, or work at some kind of menial job to survive. That really bothered me. I always wanted to read something beautiful about our people, but instead they taught us in books and on billboards, that 'Nobody loves a drunken Indian.'"

Arvol found solace and comfort in practicing his spiritual ways. He was raised with his grandmother, who taught him Lakota traditions. He also learned from the elders of the tribe, and this gave him the spiritual foundation and values to help sustain him through some very turbulent times. "As I was growing up, I remember feeling that I hoped I would always get along with everyone, because I wanted to stay humble, and respectful of all things. That was the way my grandmother taught us and she did a really good job in helping us to appreciate our tradition and way of life. She would say, 'Always have a good mind, and a good heart, because the Creator Spirit can talk to you in many different ways.' It made me happy to listen to the elders talk about our way of life. These leaders were so beautiful and powerful, because they believed in living a peaceful and harmonious life. There were so many stories shared about our traditions, and I was honored to be part of that circle. I knew that someday if people could stand up and share about our beautiful culture and traditions, I wanted to be one of them."

Dreams can be especially helpful in guiding us through life. Shortly after Arvol became Keeper of the Sacred Pipe, he had a dream that shook his world. "In the dream, I came out of the house, and the door opened itself. It was nighttime. I went up into the air, then I took a flip and I looked down, and the ground was all brown. All the grass and all the trees—and I felt like the energy was different. I told the elders the dream the next day, and they said that I would see those changes in my life." This dream helped to prepare Arvol for his life's work of creating global healing through world peace and prayer.

In 1990, at a ceremony at Wounded Knee, the elders shared with Arvol "that a black cloud would be coming after that ceremony. This black cloud was going to bring on a lot of sickness, and only the people who had a belief in their cultural ways would survive that time. People who only believe in their own back pockets, their minds would go crazy. And we would see a lot of changes start to happen, in the seventh generation, starting in 1990, that would affect the air, the water, and the land. And that we see today."

In moving through his pain, Arvol continued to heal and to grow by listening to the words of the ancient Prophecies instilled in him by the spiritual elders. It was said that there would come a time when a white buffalo calf would be born, and according to Lakota prophesy the white buffalo calf would signify a new and final chance for bringing about unity between the red, white, black, and yellow peoples. It also meant that we could choose to live according to the laws of technology or of nature. If we chose nature we would need to learn from our errors of polluting the earth and destroying life. And if we chose to live in harmony with nature, there would still be a chance for peace in the world.

The birth of the white buffalo calf in 1994 gave Arvol greater understanding of the importance of his role as a spiritual leader in helping to bring about peace and unity throughout the world. "The story told to me as a child had now come to pass, that the White Buffalo Calf Woman's spirit would make her presence known—a sign of great changes signifying the crossroads. I never dreamed I would live to witness this momentous time. White Buffalo Calf Woman's spirit has announced her message of support in this time of great danger, and she continues to announce the message in the birth of each White Buffalo—each one of them a sign, each one a fulfillment of ancient Prophecy as well as a new Prophecy for our times. We must understand the positive and negative influences that affect all life yet to come. We ourselves must make the right decision on behalf of the Seventh Generation, for our children and for their children's children."

Arvol has traveled across the globe bringing awareness of the wisdom in the ancient Lakota, Dakota, and Nakota prophecies, warning humankind of the necessity to live in peace and harmony with our Mother Earth, natural creation, and with one another. To this end, he continues to bring World Peace and Prayer Day to the Four Corners of Mother Earth, honoring sacred sites.

The first World Peace and Prayer Day ceremony was held in the Sacred Black Hills at Gray Horn Butte on June 21, 1996. Each year since Arvol has taken the ceremony elsewhere in the world. On June 21, 2001, it was held in South Africa, where one of the hosts was Gandhi, the granddaughter of Mahatma Gandhi. Says Arvol, "It is so beautiful to know that there are people all over the world who are beginning to have respect for Mother Nature, the sacred sites, the medicine, and the cultural beliefs, because we are responsible as human beings to take care of Mother Earth. She is a spirit and we are all affected by how she is treated."

Although Arvol was told by his teacher that he could never be a leader and make a difference in the world, instead of accepting those words, he chose to convert his anguish by turning to prayer, inner reflection, and ceremony. Once again he was able to listen to his heart, and to the words of the elders and of the Spirit. Today Arvol's voice, and the voice of his ancestors, remind us what it means to be a good human being, caring for each other and for all of natural creation—the true definition of success.

Chapter Three

"We're addicted to a lot of attachments that keep us from ourselves, from God, and from one another." —*Martin Sheen*

When I was growing up, I thought an addict had to be someone passed out on the street intoxicated from alcohol or another form of drug. Or that a person who had to drink or use daily was an addict. Never would I have believed that people like my father, given prescription drugs by his doctor initially to lose weight and then later to stay awake, would become dependent on these stimulants. Time and again when he took the medication he would exhibit emotional outbursts that one observes in addictive behavior. I was deeply affected by this emotional upheaval. Although my father struggled with his dependency on stimulants for some five years, I am fortunate that he chose to stop using the prescription drugs and that our family was able to begin its healing journey. I loved my father dearly. And because when he was not using he was extremely loveable and fun to be with, for many years I was attracted to men with similar qualities and habits as my father. I was accustomed to the roller-coaster, drama-filled days, and it wasn't until much later in life that I became willing to look within myself and at my life more honestly. I now know that children who are raised on drama tend to create more drama in their adult worlds. I grew to understand that being addicted refers to surrendering habitually or compulsively to something.

In my forties, I was able to recognize the pattern in my family and in myself of what addiction does not only to the addict, but the family as well. I began attending Naranon meetings that help to support the family members of addicts. Addiction brings much pain and distress to the addict and the family members of addicts. Going to Alanon and Naranon meetings was extremely helpful in my recovery. Sharing one another's stories and supporting each other in our healing makes the process of recovery more successful. On my personal healing journey, Martin Sheen, Gerald Jampolsky, Dick Gregory, Jack Canfield, and John Funmaker have each given me greater insight, inspiration, and understanding about healing and transforming the pain of addiction.

Addiction is a disease and it runs through families regardless of age, gender, and ethnicity. Martin Sheen has grown to understand the face of addiction in himself and in his family. He has also chosen recovery, and in so doing has gained tremendous wisdom and understanding from the pain he has learned to heal and transform. Martin shares, "I'm recovering from an addiction to alcohol. This is a key to my constant realization of my own weakness and my own ego, and a fault which, it seems to me, is evident in all of us to take the easy way out. We want to have our cake and eat it too."

Martin understands that we are addicted to many things. "Whether you're alcoholic or not, our addictions are manyfold. We're addicted to ourselves egotistically, we're addicted to food, images, behavior, and prejudices, not just chemical dependency. We're addicted to a lot of other attachments that keep us from ourselves, from God, and from one another."

Part of the pain of addiction is living in denial, which means we cannot admit to our innermost self that there is a problem. On Martin's healing journey he has discovered that "denial is what most of us live the majority of the time. It's not something I can talk about easily. Anybody who has been there or is there knows what it is. It is all of our worst fears confirmed. We accept responsibility for it, we reject responsibility for it; we rage, and we are humbled. We're exalted and we're cursed, we are on the mountaintop one day and deep in the valley the next. Those people who have gone through this understand what we call the roller-coaster ride. As with everyone, it's personal. Each individual is different, and there are as many levels of pain as there are people suffering from it."

Millions of people across the globe achieve sobriety participating in the twelve-step program of Alcoholics Anonymous. Martin utilized this program and has been in recovery for more than twenty years. He says, "The sole purpose of AA is to keep people sober in every spectrum of society—black, white, men, women, young, old, rich, and poor. Everyone has an equal stake in their own sobriety and the way it works is by scrupulous honesty with ourselves and service to our neighbors."

Martin was able to apply the teachings he learned in his own recovery process during his son Charlie's crises with substance abuse. Over the years they have continued to learn and grow together. Martin says, "The lessons we have both learned are still going on. We have a lot of issues that are now out in the open. The passage of time has been very healing for both of us. It's an ongoing process, you know. I adore him. He may be my greatest teacher. My wife said that about him months ago at the height of the crises, and I thought she was mad. She said, 'He's the only one who has forced us to look at ourselves and be honest with where we were, who we were, and how we were. He took us into places we never would have chosen to go on our own. That's a teacher.' We learned about the need for scrupulous honesty in our lives."

Developing faith and trust are essential to recovery. In letting go of the old and making space for the new, all things are made possible. Martin understood this when he could see that his old belief system was not working to help himself or his son, so he opened his heart and mind to the possibility of the healing coming about in a new way. Today, Martin is still in wonder at how exquisite the healing process has been. "What I have been through and how it came about, the mystery of it overwhelms me. I can only tell you this. For years I had prayed for the 'poof' miracle. You know what that is? 'Poof,' make it better. 'Poof,' God make him well. 'Poof,' God make this happen. For years this was my prayer."

A turning point for Martin was when he shifted his perception about his role in the healing process. He shares, "When I began to pray and ask God to make me part of the miracle, I got frightened and it scared me. I was afraid my prayer would be answered and I would be the 'Poof.' I would be the instrument of God's presence, and it would demand letting go of my fear and safe place, and I would have to step out into the arena and be present. I would have to confront the demons within myself and others, and I would have to tell the truth, the whole truth, nothing but the truth all the time and take the consequences. And the more I prayed, the more it became evident, that was the only way that God could help my son. And that's exactly what happened. So the scariest moment was when I realized that not only was I part of this process, but at the time, in that place, with that person, in this way, I was the only one who could do it. That is what you call the epitome of fear, the epitome of loneliness, and it is also the epitome of faith, because I didn't know in each step if the earth would remain level—yet I kept walking. That's faith. And at the end of the crises, and this horrible battle that was going on for so long, my wife and I came through still standing."

When we are ready and willing to heal, it is common to have an epiphany or revelation that helps to reassure us that the ground we are standing on is solid and that we are being Divinely guided and protected. Martin was blessed with such an experience, and this taught him the meaning of trust and faith. "During the crisis with Charlie's drug addiction, I went to a mass in downtown L.A. A friend of mine is a pastor at St. Agatha's church and I had gone there on several occasions, although I'm a member of Our Lady of Malibu. I went to this ten o'clock mass at St. Agatha's down on Adams Boulevard near La Brea, in the hood, it's a black church, a brown church, my friend is white and he's the pastor there. During this mass for the first time I relaxed and surrendered. And I felt a deeply personal Presence. And I wept with joy and relief that I had done my part in this miraculous business. I had the revelation that I was ruled by faith, that I understood fear was useless, faith was necessary, and love was everything. The clouds didn't open, I didn't hear the voice of God or thunder, I just became aware of a Presence that I know is always with me. I was quiet long enough, and it was quiet enough around me, to have this realization.

"I've been going to this community at St. Agatha's quite often since then. There is such a joyful feeling of celebration there. I was nurtured there in a way that I had not anticipated. I wept tears of great, great joy, and tears of relief, and tears of regret. But the over-all feeling was of miraculous mystery and I was part of it. It was the most gratifying reality imaginable. I cannot even describe it beyond just that. My faith had led me to a certain knowledge of God's Presence in all of this business. What can I tell ya?"

From Martin's journey in healing and transforming his pain, he was gifted with spiritual understanding that has nourished and sustained him through the most arduous and painful of times. With his faith, he has been given the insight and fortitude to, most lovingly, share with others the importance of discovering the gift in pain.

Dr. Gerry Jampolsky also sought refuge from his pain, in addiction to alcohol, until he had a spiritual awakening that guided him towards recovery and renewal.

Gerry Jampolsky, M.D., bestselling author and the founder of the

Center for Attitudinal Healing, shares, "I didn't really have any kind of transformation process until I was fifty years of age." At that time he was an alcoholic going through a very painful divorce. *"A Course in Miracles* became like my heartbeat. That was the conscious beginning of healing the pain from my childhood."

In Gerry's recovery, he began to understand the nature of his addiction and what had created it. "Alcohol was the way I drowned my pain. And the alcohol addiction was used for back pain and for emotional pain. And even after I started my spiritual journey, I continued to drink very heavily. It wasn't until after about six months that I was awakened one night by a voice speaking to me saying, 'It's no longer necessary to drink, you're in a new phase of healing.' And I thought maybe I was going into D.T.s, because it was an external voice. At any rate, I stopped drinking at that point. Then I realized I had gained a lot of weight, so I lost about thirty-five pounds the next few months. And that was a big shift for me, to let go of my weight."

Gerry learned to forgive himself, understanding that he used alcohol because he thought it would bring him relief from his suffering. He also began to forgive everyone else he was holding grudges against, because he realized we are each doing the best we can, and if we knew better, we would do better. He also came to the realization that our pain is directly connected to how spiritually connected we feel. "Much of the pain that most of us have is not just physical, but also spiritual. All pain has psychological components. Often there is guilt or grievances and unforgiving thoughts. I think that it's important for people to really take a look at their grievances and their unforgiving thoughts. We need to seek where we haven't forgiven ourselves or forgiven someone else. That is where the healing begins."

Like Gerry, Dick Gregory is a seeker of truth. He began his journey looking outside of himself for answers, and in time, began to understand that the truth lies within. Through his fasting, done with prayer and in solitude, Dick began to recognize and understand the nature of his addictions.

Many of us are not aware of our addictions, because we are of the belief that if what we consume or do is legal, then it must not be an addiction. Dick Gregory says, "I smoked four packs of cigarettes a day. I really didn't realize I was addicted to the cigarettes because as long as I could afford what I wanted, then I didn't think it was an addiction. I thought of addiction when hearing about drug dealers, when people start robbing people, and seeing the winos standing on the corner out there begging just to get a bottle."

Dick started to come out of his denial when he started to fast. He explains, "I never really understood addiction until I started fasting. When I went on my first forty-day fast I didn't consciously give up my addictions. I didn't say, 'I'm not going to smoke cigarettes again or drink alcohol again.' It's just you don't do it while you're fasting. And not smoking or drinking didn't bother me, because my number-one addiction was food. And so when you give up eating, all the other addictions leave. I never craved a cigarette or alcohol while I was on a fast. But I couldn't have anything to eat, and that was the first time I realized how powerful addiction was. We're addicted to eating from the first day of our life as though nothing else mattered."

He then began to focus on his other addictions. "I got hooked on cigarettes and alcohol because they are legal. If drugs had been legal, I would have been on them too." Dick took the time to reflect and gain greater understanding of himself and the nature of his addictions during his fast. For Dick, fasting was a saving grace that gave him a new perspective, an inner awareness, and a feeling of being connected spiritually. "I got so clean and pure from the fasting that taking my first drink of alcohol again burned my throat, and I said, 'No way!' And when I took my first cigarette again, I said, 'No way!' That's how I stopped smoking, drinking, and overeating."

Recovery is not an easy process. John Funmaker is testament to this fact. Today John is a Native American spiritual leader and drug and alcohol counselor at the Robert Sundance Wellness Center in Los Angeles, but he was an addict and alcoholic for nearly twenty years. John was born into a loving and traditional Winnebago family who spoke their indigenous language and lived according to their cultural and spiritual ways. But after being forced by the government to attend government boarding school where they were stripped of their dignity, he became angry and depressed. In his pain and confusion, turned to alcohol and drugs. John shares, "As a child I was very fortunate, being raised on the reservation in the country, and having an open space, and a lot of freedom. I had a creek to swim in and I was able to just run around. We had a few horses, and it was nice. I had a mostly positive childhood until I was nine or ten years old and I started going to school. After that I can remember only pain and confusion."

Because John was from a traditional family and he spoke very little English, other children at school who spoke better English often ridiculed him. "When I was at home I was educated in a traditional manner, with oral teachings. And I was taught about values and how we should conduct ourselves. What my parents and my family taught me was very beautiful. But I wasn't able to use what my parents had taught me in White society.

"My grandmother made me this beautiful vest of deer hide, which was something really special. This deer hide took a lot of time to prepare, and she had cut it, beaded it, and added fringe to it. It was really beautiful. She made this vest for me to wear to school, thinking that was a proper way to dress.

"But when I went to school that first day, I was ridiculed. My vest was a 'traditional' piece of clothing that was looked down upon, not only by the teachers but also by my peers. When I showed up in school wearing that vest, with my long hair in braids, I was ridiculed and punished. I don't know what the purpose was, whether to teach me a lesson, or to let my family know that my vest was not allowed at school.

"They proceeded to cut my hair, and my vest was taken off of me. After they cut my hair, I was taken down to where they had a furnace. They made me open the furnace door and put my braids in there. And they made me put the vest into the furnace as well. Those were both very sacred to me."

John says, "That kind of pain and suffering is deeper than physical pain. Today, I realize it took a lot of courage for my parents to teach me our traditional ways. But in my confusion, I became angry. Some of that anger was toward my parents, toward my own people.

I thought it wasn't good to be an Indian, because of all the ridicule of our ways. It felt like it was too hard to be Indian."

As John learned, if we do not learn how to heal our hurt, then we either turn the pain inward and become self-destructive, or we turn it outward and hurt others. "When I was growing up, I had these negative thoughts and feelings about myself. I had really poor self-esteem. I attempted suicide several times in my confusion. I didn't seem to fit in any place. Maybe that was part of my wandering. I think I crisscrossed this country several times, trying to figure something out. So by the time I ended up on skid rows and in the local jail, I was drinking and using drugs. I lived my life this way for almost twenty years. A few times I got clean and sober, only to start up drinking again."

John's use of alcohol and drugs led him to live on skid row. When he did get clean and sober he also received help from a man named Archie Fire Lame Deer, who became a spiritual teacher to him. Having a mentor and teacher can create an opening for healing and recovery from addiction. Archie Fire Lame Deer invited John to participate in some ceremonies that John used to do when he was young. When he was invited to a sweat lodge ceremony, John couldn't believe that a simple invitation could make such a difference in his life. He remembers, "Here I was in California, thousands of miles from my home. This was something I thought I was always trying to run away from, and this man invited me to come to a ceremony. So I went, partly out of curiosity. I was just wondering—is this guy for real or what is he doing? So I went and he was pretty real, and pretty traditional. Some of the songs he sang, I had heard sung before. I was in shock for a couple of months. I was kind of afraid, too, because there were a lot of painful memories in all of it. But I went and talked to Archie, and then started hanging around him. It seemed to me that he was a pretty happy man most of the time, always laughing and joking. He told me I could be Indian, and that it was okay. He gave me permission. That was the beginning of my healing. And I started meeting more people, and with them it was okay to be what I am. It felt good."

John has lost a lot of brothers and sisters to alcohol in his extended family, first and second cousins whom he grew up with. He shares, "We never had alcohol in our Indian culture before. It not only affects family, but it affects the whole community, and beyond the community. If we don't get free from our addictions, then it just goes on to the next generation. Ninety-nine percent of the people that I work with come from alcoholic homes and alcoholic families. Quite a few of them lost their parents. Either they don't know their parents, because they've been taken away from their parents and raised in other homes, or their parents died of cirrhosis of the liver or some alcohol-related problem, disease, car accident, or suicide. Alcoholism really affects everybody. It affects the whole family, it affects the next generation."

Today, John's work as a spiritual advisor and drug and alcohol counselor is in direct response to the pain he has experienced. "I work in the sweat lodge, a traditional ceremonial place of prayer, for the Native American women who are in prison. The sweat lodge is a powerful way for them to reconnect with their culture and their spirituality. In my other work as a substance abuse counselor, I see so much suffering and pain. A lot of that pain is caused from being taken away from their culture, and not being really connected to their ancestral roots and their identity." But he is dedicated to healing the gap between native people and their culture, identity, and spirituality. He says, "I understand the pain that continues when this connection is not made. There is a lot of pain and suffering among native people. I also feel hopeful and good about my work, and the work of many others who are working in the communities with their own people. There is much that needs to be done."

Growing up with the pain and insanity of addiction motivated Jack Canfield, coauthor of *Chicken Soup for the Soul*, to seek emotional, mental, and spiritual healing in his own life. He says, "I did a lot of work on my self in therapy, and I read the twelve-step books. I felt like the issues of growing up with the pain of addiction in my family were handled in my therapy. I also participated in weekend workshops, weeklong retreats, and self-help seminars, and I learned to meditate."

Jack lived with the pain of addiction for much of his life. In Jack's case, both his mother and father struggled with alcoholism. "My father was an alcoholic throughout the years he lived with us, and in his second marriage he got sober. My mother, until ten years ago, was an alcoholic, and now is sober at eighty-one. The addiction definitely ended my parents' marriage, and it certainly ended my mother's second marriage, because my stepfather got tired of it. She would drink, and then all of her repressed rage toward life and men in general would come up. And she had three sons, so we were part of the focus of that rage. That was really hurtful and caused me much pain and confusion."

Growing up with alcoholism in the family showed Jack and his siblings how destructive this disease can be. Jack shares, "In my own life, I've had periods when I drank too much, although I've never considered myself, or been labeled by anyone who's a professional, an alcoholic. But there were periods when my last marriage was not working that I would drink a half a bottle of wine with dinner. That was a way of numbing out the fact that I was really bored and lonely at night in the relationship. Today, this is not an issue in my life. Now I have a glass of wine every two weeks or so. I think drinking didn't match my self-image of health consciousness. And also, I had the ability to stop."

Jack believes he never had a problem with chemical addiction because "after drinking I felt lousy the next morning and it was not congruent with my life's purpose, which I define as inspiring and empowering people to live their highest vision in the context of love and joy. And I've always been mission driven since my mid-twenties, and I've always been very health conscious."

But it is extremely painful to recognize that although we may have learned what it means to be healthy, and to live our lives accordingly, our children still may find themselves in the throes of addiction. As did Martin Sheen, Jack Canfield faced the problem of having a son addicted to drugs. Jack remembers, "I think he suffered tremendously when I divorced his mother when he was just two years old. One of the great pains of my life is that I did not have a close relationship with my son for the first ten years of his life. His mother had moved to the West Coast and I was living on the East Coast. She was very angry at me, because I was the one who left, and so rather than continue to stay more connected, I kept busy with work to numb my pain. Today, at the age of twenty-eight, my son has been sober for some twelve months. The healing journey has not been quick nor easy, and it has been extremely painful for the entire family. He lived in a sober living house in San Francisco for a year and now lives in New York, where he attends AA meetings every day.

"The thing that helped my son the most was attending the Hoffman Quadrinity Process in San Francisco, California, which helps people clear their dysfunctional patterns in reaction to their parents. It made him 'teachable' for the first time. It released a lot of pain for him and made him available for help."

From every dark and painful experience, light and healing can emerge. About himself and his family, Jack relates, "From the agony of all of this came a most extraordinary blessing. We were told about a recovery program that is spiritually inspired. In this program, for the first time, my son has felt a connection with his higher power, and has begun to pray. This is giving him the strength and determination to begin the process of moving through and beyond the pain of addiction." Jack has been able to find the wisdom to help people cope with the many layers of pain present in families with substance abuse. The family dysfunction and ensuing hurt that substance abuse caused catapulted Jack onto a healing journey. And what Jack has learned along the way, he shares with others through his books and seminars. As Jack so poignantly illustrates, we teach best what we most need to learn.

Recovery from addiction takes people back to themselves and to their Creator. They look at what created the addiction and begin to forgive themselves and others, because they did the best they could, knowing what they knew at the time. They learn the importance of feeling their connection in order to transform their pain into healing. In time, they begin to realize that they no longer value their addictions. And in the recovery process they are able to recognize the gift of pain that can be used as a catalyst to assist them into becoming stronger, better, and wiser people.

Chapter Four

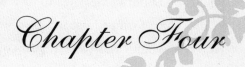

Remembering Who We Are After
Separation and Divorce

"I wish that in transforming pain people would begin to develop a less aggressive and abusive language. . . . lessons, experiences, and opportunities *as opposed to* bad relationships, broken marriages, *and* busted families.*"*

—*Iyanla Vanzant*

When two people take vows to remain together, it is a beautiful, sacred union that both parties intend on fulfilling forever. Marriage is commitment that is much more than what a piece of paper reveals. It is a bonding of heart and soul. But when a divorce or major separation happen, it can be one of the most painful occurrences in a person's life. I know this because in a period of thirty years I had two significant relationships, each ending in separation or divorce. I walked into each relationship feeling wounded and incomplete. And each time I held the belief that this man's love would make me whole. I had not yet learned to love myself.

I met my former husband Dan while living in Colombia, South America, when I was twenty years old. He was also from California and we shared many of the same concerns and views about life. Dan was Native American—Kiowa and Cherokee—and he was eager to learn about the people of the southern hemisphere. We lived in Colombia for nearly a year and then traveled by riverboat, bus, and train from Chile to Los Angeles in the course of a year. We were in Chile together during the revolution, and we learned about the rich culture and way of life of the indigenous people of Brazil, Peru, and other regions throughout South America.

We were extremely happy together, and when we returned to Los Angeles we enrolled into the University of California, Los Angeles and studied Latin American studies and public health. Dan began to identify more as an indigenous person and became active with Native American people's rights. As a Jewish person taught to stand up against injustice, I felt at home supporting native people in their struggle to regain their lands and rights. I also participated in the struggle of other people's fight for their human and civil rights. But as we stood up for what we believed, the university threatened to revoke our scholarships. And instead of becoming closer, Dan and I began to fight with each other. The pressure was too much for us. Paradoxically, although it appeared as if we were strong because people saw us as one; in truth, we were each losing our identity and pulling one another down—to the point of destroying our marriage. All of our issues of abandonment, not feeling good enough, lovable, and loved came up. We did not have the understanding, the readiness, or the willingness to heal the deep-rooted pain of our aching hearts. We ended up separating and later divorcing.

For months after our separation, I awoke each morning feeling lost and confused. At that time I would have said I was drowning in sorrow, but now I understand the power of words to define our experiences, whether they are in the present or past, and I would call this a time of grief, learning, and reorganization.

Many of us stay stuck in the pain caused by separation or divorce. We feel brokenhearted and unable to heal from the loss. It's a great challenge to learn how to live again and more important, learn how to love again. Dr. Gerald Jampolsky felt tormented and confused after his divorce. He says, "After my marriage of twenty years ended, I was filled with tremendous anger and guilt. And because of the guilt I began having a lot of back problems, and physical problems as well. I felt that the relationship would never get healed because of the degree of anger that we both had, and because we were projecting our guilt onto each other."

What often causes the most pain is not knowing how to heal yourself when the separation has occurred. Barbara Brennan, healer, therapist, and scientist, has devoted more than twenty years to research and exploration of the human energy field. Her first book, *Hands of Light,* is recognized as one of the primary texts for alternative healing in our time. She is the founder and director of the Barbara Brennan School of Healing, and her workshops, lectures, and demonstrations have taken her throughout North America, Mexico, Japan, and Europe. Barbara experienced some abuse when growing up, and her first husband was, at times, violent. She remem-bers, "I thought I should be able to move through our challenges and make them better. In time I grew to understand that this was not the right place for me to be. Part of the transition from marriage to sep-aration, and the idea of divorce, was the fact that I had to handle my traditional beliefs, which were that once I make a commitment, I keep it. No matter what. And I should be able to fix this. I learned an enormous amount from this experience because I went into the mar-riage completely naïve, and devoid of any self-knowledge. I learned a lot directly from my ex-husband, at the time I was married to him, and I learned much about my own psychodynamics. An entire world opened up for me—the world of the inner space. I don't know what my life would be like today, if I hadn't had those experiences."

Over time, the pattern of being abused as a child by her father and as an adult by her husband became clear to Barbara. "In the begin-ning, I walked into his family, totally naïve, and suddenly all of this violence came up. I had not had any abuse since those few years of childhood. When I started to get abused again after I got married, all the memories of abuse I had received as a child in my family came up. I knew it was time for me to work on that. I was in years of ther-apy, couple sessions, and family sessions, we were in groups with other couples. We worked, and worked as much as we could on it. Most of my time was focused on working out those abuse issues, or being in the middle of them." Barbara shares that "essentially, we were stand-ins for each other's shadow self. Or lower self, depending on which language you use for that. That shadow is for the negative unconscious. Essentially we stood in for each other. And from this, I had to face my own fears. I had to face my issues, I had to claim my life."

A turning point for Barbara was when she was living in a spiritual community, and although the abuse was much less but still ongoing, she continued to have numerous psychic experiences. She says, "I was seeing auras and was very sensitive to energy. I decided to go to Los Angeles to a healing workshop and to have some private healings. I went through fifteen past lifetimes in a week and a half. This was in the early '70s. And in every one of them, I saw myself having the same pattern. It was curious. There were fifteen lifetimes, I had been married fifteen years. And there were fifteen different patterns. I had gotten killed or died from each pattern, in each of the fifteen lifetimes. I knew this was a warning and that I was headed toward another death."

Barbara decided to get one more reading to be absolutely clear. "The reader told me I was ten years behind my life's task! By this time I was a path-work helper, a bioenergetic therapist, and a core helper. And the dynamic had softened because I had learned how not to get beaten up by this guy. I just didn't get near him." Often when we are making a major transformation, our body goes into a physical healing crisis. Barbara shares, "I got a really high fever, and I was having hallucinations for three or four days. The fever was between 104 and 105. My friend took care of me. At the time I was not aware of how many days had passed. When I got well and flew back to the East Coast I left my marriage the next day. I knew I had to leave if I wanted to survive."

Barbara became aligned with who she is and what she is here to do and she was supported by the universe. Within three months Barbara's therapy practice in New York City turned into a healing practice. She got fifty new clients. Her whole world shifted. She also invested energy in learning how to support her new way of being connected.

Barbara had a deep communion with nature, knowledge, curiosity, and beauty. In this regard, she has always experienced much inner peace. The more challenging and painful areas of her life were in relationships with people. "It was in being in relationships with human beings, intimate relationships with human beings, where I was having challenges as most of us do. That is really the deep issue for all of us. On the earth plane, the incarnation process is a learning relationship, because what we learn in relationship is love and connection, in an imperfect world. It's a lot easier to love in a perfect world."

I ADMIRE Barbara Brennan for her growth in personal relationships, and her example helps me to recognize my own process. In hindsight, I now recognize that as a twenty-year-old, I had not learned how to love myself and I did not know myself. I went into my relationship with Dan with a very fragile sense of self. He was my first great love, and I grew tremendously in the relationship. But when it ended after seven years, I fell apart. It took me nearly five years to heal and to redefine who I was. Although I was devastated by the divorce, it catapulted me into an inner search and understanding of myself. Much of that learning and growth took place in Native

American ceremonies with Medicine Men and Medicine Women. In time, my focus in life became more spiritual than political.

From this relationship I learned about the importance of being honest with myself and, with this understanding, how to be honest with others. I also learned that it was not my place to try to change my husband, and that in reality one only changes when one is ready and willing. The only person I could change was myself. It became apparent that two people with low self-esteem can bring one another down. And I grew to realize that in order for a relationship to endure and to last a lifetime, it helps to have some form of spiritual foundation. In my marriage, when we were faced with challenges, we did not know how to go within ourselves and discover the resources and connection we have to our higher power for guidance and understanding. We also did not have the tools to forgive ourselves and each other for all the pain we had caused.

I have realized that forgiveness is an essential key to all healing. And it is especially challenging when facing the breakup of a marriage because anger, fear, resentment, and all the unpleasant feelings can block any sense of compassion for the self or the other person. Rabbi Zalman Schachter is founder of the Jewish Renewal and the Spiritual Eldering Institute. He was also the past holder of the World Wisdom chair at Naropa University, where he is currently a professor. He believes the most important thing to learn is forgiveness. He says, "If you want to remain a victim, you can reinforce your victimness and the evil of the other person, and you can look around for whom you can tell your story of 'poor me.' If you want to live with that drama, you can, but it drains energy from the body and it takes away courage from the future. Forgiveness of self and forgiveness of the other person are hooked together. I can't say that I forgive the other person and then blame myself, because I can't stay in self-blame for long without blaming the other person again. There's a certain kind of mutuality in forgiveness."

In his own healing from his divorce, Rabbi Zalman was able to realize that "people grow; however, they don't necessarily grow in the same direction. The tension between two people may get to be so great that it feels as if it cannot be calmed. But that is something you have to work on, and that is extremely important in divorce issues. What you're divorcing is the spousal relationship. But the co-parenting relationship you never divorce. You really need to collaborate, and there can be a lot of goodwill in collaborating. My ex-wife and I learned how important that was, and when it came time to stand together at the altar when our children got married, we had a lot of goodwill toward one another."

He also believes that having an emotional foundation is essential when moving through a divorce: "In a divorce you can have an emotional foundation that says, 'I do remember that I was loved. I do remember that I could love. I do remember that I acted decently, and I do remember that I am an altruistic person most of the time.' You can remember the strengths and the gifts of the relationship."

The turning point for Gerry Jampolsky was when he became a student of *A Course in Miracles*. He says, "I began to see the power of forgiveness. Miracles began to happen, and today my relationship with Pat, my ex-wife, is beautiful. We're very close, we spend time with the kids together and at Thanksgiving, Christmas, Halloween, and other special occasions. We are supportive of each other, and I've learned that the pain of an unhappy marriage is relieved when we forgive ourselves and forgive others. I had to realize that my ego did not want to forgive myself or anyone else. I became more committed to asking for God's help along the way. This kind of commitment makes things happen. This progress was a gradual thing and is a continual process."

Gerry began to realize that if you're hurting someone else, you're also hurting yourself. As he explains, "I think everyone is our Siamese twin. So everyone's our soulmate in that sense of the word. And I began to realize that what I was seeing in her that I didn't like was something also in myself. So in the end I was healing myself and my relationship with God, letting go of my fear of God, and realizing that God will always keep me covered. Having trust and faith in God is the core to this kind of shift in perception."

Gerry's second wife, Diane Cirincione, says that her first marriage did not honor her authentic self. "My first marriage was radically opposed to who I was. We were trapping and fishing and hunting. My first husband's brothers were all hunters and he was too. I forced myself to be involved with my husband's life, and I learned to fish and hunt. I had to really numb my own feelings to become involved with my husband's activities. I thought I was supposed to do that.

"And I remember we were walking in the woods in Northern California at one time and we saw this giant white heron. I had never seen a heron, and I was so awestruck by its beauty, watching it flying above us in slow motion with its six-foot wingspan. And someone in the group pulled his gun up and shot this heron out of the sky. And it fell. I remember being so shaken by the experience. And of course my husband was upset, and other people were upset too, but I remember looking at the bird and looking around me and thinking, 'I'm out of here.'

"Even though I didn't say it out loud at the time, I knew in my mind I was going. I thought, 'You are so out of who you are, out of integrity with who you are.' Now I'm grateful of the experience of my first marriage because it helped me to dispel the illusions I had about myself, to discover my authentic self, and to strengthen and honor my individuality."

After her divorce she chose to learn about who she is and what she wanted out of life. This helped her to create a relationship that would honor and nurture her true nature. Diane shares, "In this relationship with Gerry, we were both single seventeen years before we married. That wasn't by accident! We knew each other nine and a half years before we married. And for me, a part of that was to be really clear about finding out who I was, and being cognizant about my own identity and boundaries before I could even look at being in a relationship with someone who is as strong and clear as Gerry is. And it wasn't a day too soon. It was just perfect."

Perhaps forgiveness is most difficult when coming out of an abusive marriage. Millions of women throughout the world are in emotionally and physically abusive relationships, and yet they don't leave because they either fear for their lives or don't feel they could make it on their own. In an abusive relationship, perhaps more than at any other time, it is of utmost importance to be able to listen to guidance from within and to stay spiritually connected. Best-selling author Iyanla Vanzant left a physically abusive marriage and today she empowers men and women all over the world with her books, teachings, and outreach. Like so many, it took her a long time to reach an understanding about forgiveness.

"I was in an abusive marriage," she says, "and something woke me up out of my sleep and said, if you don't leave here, he's gonna kill you. When I say 'something' I literally mean *something*, because I didn't have a clue. There was nothing to be seen, nothing . . . I didn't argue, I didn't fight, I was literally told step by step what to do. 'Get up, don't go over there, you don't need that, take this, take that, get the kids, wake up your son first.' I was told everything I was to do, and I followed it. It wasn't until I got to the train station at five o'clock in the morning with these three babies that I said, 'I haven't got a clue as to where I'm going.' I started walking back towards the house and the presence said, 'No, get on the train and go there, go there, go.' So, I think that was the time when I first became consciously aware that there was really truly a power that will guide you and heal you and it wasn't until I got out of my marriage and began doing other things that I realized how painful being in that marriage was. When I was there I thought, 'I can't leave, where can I go, I've got three kids, there's no place I can go.' But then I got out and I went to college, I met other people and I began to heal my pain."

In taking time to reflect and seek understanding, Iyanla began to recognize that "when I was on welfare, all my friends were on welfare; when I was in confusion, all my friends were in confusion—

misery really does love company. And that's what makes the misery so normal to you, 'cause everybody had it. When I think of things that I just accepted as normal, it scares me. It's amazing to me today. I began to see the truth in this some twenty-five years ago."

Iyanla grew into becoming honest with herself and to understand the truth about who she is and what had happened in her relationships. She remembers, "I was still mad. I had to ask myself, what was I mad at? What I was really mad at was myself. I was mad that I had stayed that long; I was mad that I had accepted the abuse, because my marriage was a very abusive marriage. I was angry that I couldn't get him to do what I wanted him to do. I was angry that he left me for another woman. And I was angry that, while he was abusing me and sleeping around, I stayed. That's what I was angry at, but of course I put that on him. So once I really could sit down with myself and tell the truth about what really happened, and accept my share of the responsibility for what went on, and how long it went on, then I could begin to move out of the pain."

The moment that we own up to our own responsibility in the relationship and look honestly at our own behavior is when we can begin to forgive. Iyanla shares, "Instead of being angry with him, I had to learn to forgive myself for thinking I had done anything wrong. I had to learn to forgive him for thinking he had, and I had to learn to forgive myself for thinking he had done anything wrong. What I recognized is that we all do the best we can, and the minute we know better, we'll do better. No matter how ugly, no matter how painful, no matter what it looks like, we all do the best we can. And for me, moving out of that pain was what I wanted to do, but I had to tell the truth about it."

Often, pain pushes and vision pulls us toward what we need. My second deep relationship that lasted for sixteen years was a bitter-sweet love, filled with much soulful connection, passion, and a shared need to work for just causes. However, we did not have a spiritual foundation together, and eventually he began to have affairs. Honesty, trust, and commitment began to erode. There were many apologies and promises, but without the readiness to heal, basically the same theme remained throughout our years of entering and leaving one another's lives. It was particularly painful, because we were not the only two people involved in this relationship. Our daughter, Imani, has had to endure and to grow from all of our mistakes.

In this relationship there was abuse, lack of respect, and infidelity that manifested in my being unhappy and physically ill. I had a nervous stomach, was often unsettled, anxious, moody, angry, hurt, resentful, wanting to focus on him and what was wrong with him, and at times not focusing on my daughter. I began to realize that I was allowing this man's life to run mine, since my focus was on him. I felt sad, angry, and ashamed with myself that I had given so much of my life and power to him. I felt that I went terribly astray in living my life in a way that I knew was not healthy and loving toward myself and others.

I learned to be more honest with myself and feel my feelings and express them through talking with friends, praying, listening in meditation and silence, writing, dancing, music, and walking in nature. By doing these things I could remember who I was and feel my loving self. In dance I began to feel my spirit soar once again. I began to remember and create joyful moments and it became clear to me that I was in an abusive relationship. I felt as if I had sold myself out for the illusion that I would be loved, cherished, and cared for. In reality, I was not giving that to myself and in turn making healthy choices that would attract the right life mate into my life.

For Iyanla, the pain pushed her toward prayer, and prayer created an opening for the inspiration and guidance she needed to come through. She learned to move out of the way and allow this assistance to move through her. And it was with prayer that she was guided and given the strength to convert her pain. According to Iyanla, "If you pray long and hard enough, you'll get the answer. And I was praying long enough and hard enough for release from the pain. Then the answers began to flow, but I resisted them, I rejected them. I said, 'No that's not it,' and I kept blaming him, and blaming him wasn't making me feel any better." And then Iyanla was introduced to the mind-altering philosophies of Science of Mind and Unity, and writers such as Ken Keyes, Swami Muktananda, Joel Goldsmith, and Catherine Ponder. "I think the two books that had the greatest impact on me were Catherine Ponder's *The Dynamic Laws of Prayer* and Joel Goldsmith's *Practicing the Presence*. Those were my first life-aid kits."

In healing and converting her pain, Iyanla began to perceive of her "broken hearts" in a new way. She came to the realization that "my fantasy broken hearts were when my relationships didn't work out the way I wanted them to or my marriage didn't work out the way I thought it was going to. Those relationships resulted in broken hearts. The reason we're brokenhearted is because we think we're alone. He's gone. I'm alone. But we're still connected. Personally, I like the terms *lessons, experiences,* and *opportunities* as opposed to calling them *bad relationships, broken marriages,* and *busted families.*" From this Iyanla learned that we are all here to heal, and not here to fix and change one another. Acceptance is necessary rather than judgment, so when we stop judging, life unfolds differently.

She also learned how to ask the appropriate questions that would make healing possible after experiencing separation and divorce. She shares, "If we tell the truth and examine what is the purpose of this relationship, are we still on that purpose? And is the pursuit of the purpose making everybody happy?, then we will be very clear and honest with ourselves and our significant other. It's all about being happy and being truthful. If it is not working, can we accept that this isn't working? Can we accept that without blame, can we accept that and not be angry because our fantasy again was shattered? And once we get to the point where we realize we're off purpose, this isn't working, and we accept that, then are we willing to do what's necessary to keep the love and move forward even if in separate directions? Am I willing to love you even though I can't live with you? Am I willing to hold up my responsibilities to my children, to my wife or my husband, even though we're not going to be together? Am I willing to do those things? And I think if we have the truth and we have acceptance and we have willingness, the next thing is trusting the process, that as this separation unfolds, everybody is going to get what they need, exactly as they need it."

Iyanla teaches us to take the action that is needed, while trusting we will be helped. When I left my relationship, I learned about leaving the past behind as well. But I also learned how to feel the pain to the best of my ability and then heal and transform it so I could perceive what had happened in a new light. Much pain is caused by obsessing about the past or fretting about the future. What I've come to realize was that this relationship acted as a catalyst for helping me to discover who I am, and it helped create a closer relationship with my Higher Power. And, most important, it taught me to finally learn how to love myself. In doing so, I am discovering wholeness within and cherishing the recognition that my daughter and myself are enough—we are family. It has become clear that until we move through our pain, and heal, our unlearned lessons become issues that drive us throughout our lives.

When we learn and grow from our pain, it is possible to attract a mate with whom we can have a healthy and loving relationship. In Rabbi Zalman's experience, he says, "Everything changes when you have a good relationship. Thank God I have a wonderful, blissful relationship with my wife. That in itself heals much of the pain." For Goldie Hawn, her relationship with fellow actor Kurt Russell has been sustained by Goldie's understanding that she not lose herself in a relationship and that she needs to carry forth her own dreams. She explains, "We all expect our mates to share everything with us. And I think the key here is to sort of bless them for being who they are. We have a tendency to become very sad when their dreams don't

have anything to do with ours. Or let's say one person is more spiritually inclined than the other one. Sometimes these kinds of relationships sort of go by the wayside. This is very unfortunate because
to live your spiritual life, it's very personal. You don't have to take
someone's else's dreams and make them your own."

Relationships are a way to constantly discover new things about
ourselves, because our communication with our partner depends
upon knowing what we need and voicing these needs. Rickie Byars-
Beckwith is a composer and singer and the music director of the
Agape International Choir, at the Agape International Spiritual Center, in Culver City, California. Her marriage to Reverend Michael
Beckwith has been an opportunity for her to seek a true understanding of herself. Rickie shares, "Once I married a man who was a very
nice person on the one hand, but I didn't know him long enough to
know what his flight patterns were. Because it's all about how people
move. When you're flowing one way, which is your way of freedom,
and your partner says, 'No, that way doesn't work, why don't you
try this way,' they're making the judgment that it doesn't work, and
they're saying, 'Do it my way.' And before you know it you are saying, 'OK,' and leaving behind your vision of how to live your life."

She had to learn how to speak up for herself and to ask for what
she wants and needs. She says, "Now I speak out from my heart. If
something is hurting me, I say, 'This doesn't feel so good, can you
help me with this?' And that allows him to say, 'Oh, I didn't realize
that I did that.' And I can say what that made me feel like and then
he can say, 'I would never want to make you feel like that.' And I can
say, 'You may not be aware of it but this is the way you do things

sometimes. But that is really funny to me because I know that is not who you really are,' and we get to talk about it. When we can talk it out, we can be clear and we don't have to suppress our feelings." Through the healing, Rickie is becoming more complete as an individual while also learning to live in a union with her husband.

We are each on a very sacred journey. People and situations come into our lives because they allow us the opportunity to grow into the whole person we truly are. When we experience violence and abuse, it is possible to find peace and kindness instead.

Chapter Five

Restoring Harmony Between the Mind
and Body

"God does the healing, and we can be the catalyst. We need to replace the belief that 'there is nothing I can do' with the belief that 'we can make a big difference.' " —Miriam Lynette

*I*n a quiet voice, Mom phoned to tell me she was diagnosed with colon cancer. I was shocked and afraid—she was the pillar of our family, and I looked to her for strength and guidance. Mom knew how to take care of her body by doing yoga and running three times a week, and she was always interested in healthy nutrition. But like most westerners Mom's focus was always on the physical, and she did not see a connection between her emotions and her body. Feeling her emotions and moving through the pain was not what she was taught or comfortable with. Her husband, her mother, and her father all died within three years' time, and the way she coped with the loss and pain was to keep busy. And in that whirlwind she would act as if everything were fine, even when it was not.

My mom needed to not only heal her colon cancer but also her separation between her physical self and her emotional/spiritual self. It was a challenge for her to look honestly at herself and communicate her feelings. But as odd as it may sound, her experience of dying from cancer was part of what helped my mother to become open and to recognize how she had always repressed her feelings. Before she passed on, she was able to recognize that she had been pushing her feelings down to the point of being in denial, something which she felt contributed to her being ill.

Historically, our Western culture has tended to separate the mind and body into two distinct areas. In traditional medicine, the prevalent thought has been to treat "pain" by finding the physical root cause. For example, if someone has a sore throat, the explanation, according to a traditional M.D., would be that the patient has contracted a virus or has inhaled something to irritate the throat. In the mind-body area, the explanation might go beyond the physical by explaining that the patient is perhaps not communicating what they need to be saying. Perhaps they aren't speaking up in a relationship or a work situation. In other words, our thoughts and feelings affect our physical self. The mind-body health philosophy doesn't discount actual medical science, it just looks deeper and embraces a larger body of thought. In the last fifteen years, alternative medicine has rapidly been embraced by the mainstream, and today we are making new gains in this field.

One pioneer in the mind-body health movement has been Larry

Dossey, M.D., former chief of staff at Medical City Dallas Hospital. He is also the *New York Times* best-selling author of *Healing Words* and *Reinventing Medicine Health Beyond the Body.* He is an internationally esteemed speaker on spirituality and medicine and is the executive editor of the peer-reviewed journal *Alternative Therapies in Health and Medicine.*

Dr. Dossey was introduced to alternative healing in the early seventies while suffering from severe migraine headaches that caused him partial blindness, nausea, vomiting, and such severe pain that he almost dropped out of medical school. He explored biofeedback to help ease the pain, and his headaches virtually disappeared. Biofeedback uses imagery and visualization and relaxation tools to help change your physiology. At that point in his life, he wasn't aware of any mind-body connection and it completely revolutionized the way he practiced medicine. He says, "I was a typical type A individual, driven by the clock, and I was completely unaware that these mind-body events, which everyone takes for granted today, were going on. So this was a revelation for me, and it literally changed my life as a physician.

I became certified in teaching biofeedback imagery and visualization. I established a biofeedback laboratory in my own practice, which was a group practice of almost a couple dozen internists and sub-specialists, and that began an interest in my life in mind-body medicine—behavioral medicine. I followed all the research that was coming down the pipeline at that point and became somewhat of an authority in those areas. That really redirected my life, and the position that I am in at this stage in my life is a direct result from those early interests. None of that would have happened without a confrontation with pain."

Larry Dossey describes pain as "separation from our true nature. Our disconnection with the Divine. This is the most tragic example of separation in modern life. All other forms of separation pale in comparison to this, whether separation from family, homeland, loved ones, or self."

What Larry has discovered in his work is that, "We know that hope and belief and meaning and the sense of trust and faith exert tremendously potent influences on health and illness. Their results can be dramatic; they can make the difference between life and death."

Larry saw striking proof of this during his first year in practice when he treated a patient who had cancer throughout both lungs. "He was dying, he was in his seventies, he wanted me to simply discharge him to go home and die. He refused all therapy. So I did send him home. The only therapy that he had, if you want to call it that, was the congregation from his church, who came and prayed for him nonstop while he was in the hospital. I wasn't impressed with that, so I just discharged him. I expected he would die days later. But a year later one of my colleagues called me up and said, 'You know you oughta drop by and see your old patient, he's back in the hospital with a bad case of the flu.' I went down to the radiology department to look at his current chest X ray, and there wasn't any sign of cancer. The lungs were perfectly clear, compared to the old X ray that was filled with cancer. This is one of those so-called 'miracle cures.' This man had no therapy except the activation of his own faith and belief and the prayers of other people. I don't find it very interesting to argue whether or not this was really a miracle or whether something physical happened. I think those are dead-end arguments. The fact is that this was a majestic, wonderful, completely unexpected, and totally unpredictable event—a man who had two feet in the grave and got completely well."

If we're going to understand the transforming powers of pain and the discomfort and unpleasantness in general in our lives, Larry believes that "we're going to have to engage it. This generally means ceasing to act automatically. For example, instead of taking a medication to eradicate pain in the next five minutes, perhaps to sit and be with it and to explore it, to engage it psychologically and mentally for a while before doing whatever is necessary to dull the pain. It means trying to achieve a friendlier relationship with discomfort in general, toward challenges in general, of which pain is only one particular variety. It means to stop being driven by discomfort, by pain, by any sort of challenge, and try to put ourselves in the driver's seat, to have pain react to us. We don't want to be the victim of pain, but we want to listen to its messages."

He suggests one way to deal with pain is to use the particular imagery process of focusing on pain as a red ball. He explains, "To enter the pain, assign it a color, perhaps a taste, texture, shape, a round form. And after you've focused on it as intently as possible, honor that red ball as being your pain, put it in your hand, and then take that pain, that red ball of pain, and go bury it under the biggest boulder you can imagine up on a mountain, so deeply that it cannot escape. And then bow, honor, and walk back down the mountain leaving it behind. One can play these sorts of images and visualizations end-lessly and be very inventive and creative. You don't have to respond against the pain in a combative warlike mode."

He also suggests to try to not respond automatically to the pain. He says, "I try to understand it. I've learned enough to at least ask some questions before moving to separate myself from the pain. 'What's the cause of the pain? Is there a hidden meaning to this pain? Is there a lesson to be learned? Do I contribute to this in ways that I don't see? What can I learn from this? And how can I get rid of it?'"

Physical pain can be a way for us to learn how to create our life. It enables us to focus on issues that we might otherwise ignore. Barbara Brennan is a healer, therapist, and scientist who has devoted more than twenty years to research and exploration of the human energy field. In explaining her work in the energy field Barbara says, "Our physical bodies exist within a larger 'body,' a human energy field or aura, which is the vehicle through which we create our experience of reality, including health and illness. It is through this energy field that we have the power to heal ourselves. This energy body, only recently verified by scientists but long known to healers and mystics, is the starting point of all illness. Here, our most powerful and profound human interactions take place, the precursor and healer, of all physiological and emotional disturbances."

Barbara believes that our thoughts form energy blocks in our field that are a result of our family heritage. She says, "There are ways to unravel it. It's just very, very difficult. And what's difficult is that all of these energy consciousness blocks are within us. And when we're raised, we're taught how to be. And that family heritage becomes a defense system. And so we carry not only the negative or false beliefs, about how reality is, but we carry all of the defenses that protect these beliefs. We are taught to be that way."

For Barbara, healing takes place in how you respond to what another person does in interaction with you. She explains, "It is a retraining. First you find what the pain was, you feel that pain, and then you learn a healthy response to it rather than perpetuating the negative reaction that keeps it going. And all of this can be seen in the energy field, and we work directly with the energy field as well as these concepts."

She adds, "An effective way I know of healing pain is to understand the difference between the pain of resistance and the pain of surrendering to the truth of what is." This requires a tremendous amount of willingness to receive information that may seem foreign. In converting our pain, Barbara understands that "it is important to surrender to the truth of what really was and what is right now. And experience that. It doesn't mean that you will surrender to and then be in pain forever. It means softening the pain, and then you are carried by that pain into your soft, loving nature. And your compassion and understanding flows up from within you automatically." What Barbara has grown to understand is that, "The pain in our life is to teach us a better way to create our life. It is also to get our attention."

Dr. Linda Fickes, another energy worker and chiropractor in Hawaii, first looks at a person's energy field and focuses on where there is a lack of life force and where there is a lack of love. She says, "I both see and feel the amount of life force in the body. I see some areas that are a little darker, or a little brighter, and what's not flow-ing. I look at and get a sense of permission, how much healing do they really want? Are they really willing? How far are they willing to go with expanding to more life force and more love? Then I look at specific symptoms and reasons why that person came into the of-fice. If the liver comes up there might be a chemical problem with liver function that needs balancing. Perhaps the person needs a nu-tritional analysis or supplements. But then as we proceed, we might find that maybe there is a thought form that's involved with the liver's dysfunction that might have to do with a resentment from childhood. This would be typical with the liver."

Linda has discovered that "we need to be most open to receiving Big Self, who we really are, what our purposes are. Through inter-acting with that energy, that is where we find our health—whether it's in our relationships, or in the simplest life activities like driving our kids to school or walking the dog. The more that we are present and breathing that energy, that is health. And where we are not do-ing that is where we find our disease." Linda reminds us to enlarge our awareness of our Greater Self that dwells above the limited and distorted teaching that obscure our full potential and our true har-monious goodness.

Miriam Lynette, life coach, healer, and mentor in Santa Fe, is a wonderful example of how generously life works for our healing and highest good when we are prepared to receive its many blessings. Lynette has transformed several of her health challenges, including a ruptured disc in her neck, by using natural health methods, and sometimes by receiving miraculous interventions.

One evening several years ago, Lynette heard a loud sound like a high volume of rushing water under pressure. At first she thought a water main had burst under the house, but in fact the sound was coming from a blood vessel in her head. She experimented with head positions to reduce the pressure, and slept sitting up.

That weekend a dear friend took her, on a impulse, to a reservation in the mountains where preparations were being made for a sweat lodge ceremony. Soon a dusty caravan of cars and trucks came winding between the trees lining the dirt road into the reservation, and an impressive Navaho Medicine Man, Hank Bainbridge, alighted and walked over to confer with the tribal leader. Then they both walked directly over to Lynette, and the leader stated, "You have a problem inside your head." Hank added, "You enter the sweat lodge after me." This meant, unknown to Lynette, that the ceremony would be dedicated to her healing.

Although Lynette realized that the intense heat of the ceremony would be risky with her condition, she made up her mind to participate, regardless. After the sacred sweat lodge ceremony she never again had a blood vessel crisis in her head. Later she heard that Hank had been leading healing ceremonies in Tuolome Meadows in Northern California that day, when spiritual guidance told him to break camp and drive down to Southern California to help heal Lynette at the reservation.

Lynette has learned from her experiences that connection and collaboration are at the core of healing and well-being. She says that "the powerful connection to activate is with the parts of the person that have been latently helpful and now need to be dominant. I believe in and lend power to the side of the person who thinks healthy and has no reason to be unhealthy."

Lynette has come to believe that Will, Belief, Intention, Emotion, Choice, and Knowing are among our greatest powers. And knowing that God does the healing and we can be the catalyst. She says, "I know that the person is connected to God and God can do anything. Disciplining the mind, using tools, and confident assumption that this will change the person's state—all are effective. Prayer, reframing, energy transfer, imagery, parables, full breathing, sound therapy, Vital Force therapy, toning, choosing archetypes, and focused intention all help the person to take charge of their well-being."

Lynette emphasizes that "all of us need to listen to each other with compassion. We need to hear beyond what is said, to hear what is really being expressed, with understanding. We need to see with compassion and love, beyond the stuck energy. We need to replace the belief that 'there is nothing I can do' with the belief that we can make a big difference. We need to take action against our inaction.

"People can be bedazzled by their limiting beliefs and disbeliefs, by their storms and inner conflicts. A healer can lend strength to a person's more positive powerful inner forces. I may sit beside someone and talk about nutrition, but what I am really doing is helping to activate their inner wellness resources. And my knowing that God is in charge and that chaos does not reign helps others to know this also. I love to connect with people who are collaborating with their spiritual power and choosing the better path."

Lynette's healing journey began with the intent to seek her own healing, and in the process she was able to discover her gifts as a healer. Lynette is a wonderful inspiration, reminding us to never leave a leaf unturned, and to embrace the infinite possibilities with which the universe blesses us.

When my mother started to open up to the connection between her repressed feelings and her cancer, we began a new phase of healing, open to the multitude of possibilities that are available in the universe. Now rather than using only conventional methods for healing, we researched alternative healing modalities to strengthen her immune system. This also required her to look more honestly at herself and recognize and release pain that had been stored for years and years. Sometimes we read about a healing way or a healer, other times we were guided to the right place at the right time and were introduced to a healing modality, and still at other times, I was guided to the next step through dreams. Sometimes she became terribly fearful and she reverted back to her Western ways of shutting down, but as they began to fail her, she searched within her heart and soul and found the faith to move forward, putting forth the best effort to heal herself.

Kahu O Te Range, a Maori Kahuna from New Zealand describes pain as "the awareness of an ending of an understanding. It's like we have to work our way through what it is that caused the pain, and acknowledge it, encompass, feel it, cry with it, laugh with it, and then release it. That's basically the Polynesian approach. We do the same thing with memories that one may perceive as being negative. Because in order to truly understand that we have to encompass it, we have to breathe it, we have to feel it, and let it resonate within our being, resonate within the cells of our being, and really feel what it feels like. And then release it.

"So it's like tasting it. It's the idea of the subjective approach. You have an incomplete experience of it until you've tasted the reality of it. But we go through life experiencing without really experiencing the experience. All we are aware of is the pain, not the experience. So the idea is to recall the experience in order to understand the pain, and in understanding the pain, having the capacity to let it go."

For Kahu, the question is, why are we here? He says, "We're here basically to remember who we are and why we're here. Since the Divine spark of God is within all things and all beings, that's why we come to this place, to remember the Divine plan. To grow through understanding, to grow through the encompassment of all things, and to express the Divinity of the Creator. To have compassion for all things, and that's what—unconditional love is, nothing more than compassion for all things, and the right of all things to exist."

Kahu believes that we are also the vehicles of our ancestors. "We are the living faces of our ancestors, so in Polynesia we might say 'We understand the principle of reincarnation.' What our ancestors did not achieve, through forgiveness, through love, through understanding, the genetic DNA memory can heal by the acknowledgment that one member of a family remembers the divine plan, and in such a way heals that memory. Heals it not only from the past but heals it for the future, so that the children born will not be born with that genetic defect."

Stephen Lewis, cofounder of the Energetic Matrix Church of Consciousness, also known as EMC^2, and co-author of *Sanctuary*, works to provide the sacrament of energetic balancing—a spiritual technology to assist in removing energetic imbalances in order to increase the life force and consciousness of living beings. He firmly believes that healing is the responsibility of the sufferer. He says, "Healing is definitively in the realm of spirituality and must be done by you. Healers don't actually heal you, but rather teach or inspire. The work is done by your consciousness directing your life force." Stephen used to be an acupuncturist and homeopathic doctor but came to recognize that imbalances first exist in the consciousness. He says, "With that consideration, I felt it was no longer appropriate for me to be in practice with patients, but instead to focus on the realm of spirituality."

Stephen adds, "More than a century after Einstein first described the energetic unity of the world, we are finally beginning to understand the spiritual and mystical implications of his discovery. There are miraculous possibilities that emerge when we view the universe as the spiritual manifestation of our unitive consciousness. Our thought gives the wave that is life particulate status. It gives it mass, it gives it form, it gives it material form. You create life with your mind. Consciousness creates matter, and consciousness can shape and change anything. And that is the fundamental message, and consciousness cannot be removed from spirituality or from healing."

One example of miraculous possibilities that can occur when we're awake to realizing the importance of our own consciousness comes from Dr. Tobin Watkinson, who understands the meaning of energy medicine. He is a nutritionist, chiropractor, acupuncturist, and psychologist who has sought out greater knowledge to be able to effectively help his patients and himself. After a bite from a brown recluse spider left him partially paralyzed and in excruciating pain, he was motivated to seek out greater knowledge about the nature of healing. After going to some doctors, Dr. Watkinson realized that they could do nothing for him. Eventually, through his friend, Dr. Margaret Ayers, he found a doctor who had brown recluse spider venom. He embarked on a course of treatment that desensitized him to the spider. Within a short period of time he was able to move, but was electrically dead from his solar plexus to his knees.

Dr. Watkinson couldn't be on his feet for long periods of time and still felt great amounts of pain. During this time he constantly asked himself why he was having this experience. He remembers, "I'm looking through the Bible for phrases of near miss, I'm reading Native American stuff on what the spider really means. And so I said, I need to get more primitive than the venom itself. Because the venom was really working as a virus, it had a life of its own. And I figured that if I got older than the venom, if I got more primitive than the venom, that I could in fact, be able to determine how I might be able to destroy the venom, or at least cause the venom to not affect me in the way it had affected me. And so I said, what's more primitive than the spider . . . it's probably electricity. And so what I needed to do is to create some sort of an electrical environment, in which my own electric could turn back on again."

So Dr. Watkinson started exploring electrical energy as a way to heal himself. He was successful and he continued to explore this field. He eventually came across a man named Ibrahim Karim, who developed a whole area of science called biogeometry. Dr. Watkinson explains, "In biogeometry they're basically using shapes that actually generate a frequency, an energy."

Dr. Watkinson went on to find disease represents the body's inability to stay tuned into, like a radio station, the frequency of health. Each organ system of the body has a resident frequency on which it operates. This resident frequency represents the health of the organ. A healthy organ has a frequency which may represent a 180-degree shift in frequency as compared to a diseased organ.

Many of us have had the experience of driving cross country. We find a great song on the radio in the middle of Kansas just as the station is overtaken by a stronger signal. The same kind of effect, Dr. Watkinson feels, occurs as the frequency of disease takes over when the frequency of health is weak. Much of Dr. Watkinson's work today is focused upon understanding the relationship between body frequency abnormalities and health.

Aside from focusing on the physical, meditation and prayer are powerful ways to heal pain. Reverend Michael Beckwith, founder of Agape International Center in Culver City, understands the importance of prayer and mediation for inner healing as well as global healing. Reverend Michael shares, "Through developing a spiritual practice of prayer and meditation, the 'unseen world' begins to be more real to you than the 'seen' world. The qualities of love, peace, and harmony begin to be more real than the transitory experiences that seem to be happening all around you. At some point you begin to become aware that you are really surrounded by spiritual ideas and not just by things. The things of the world represent ideas. You become in tune with the ideas that are fueling you." He believes that we have gathered beliefs that Jung described as "biological codings" passed down from our ancestors. And so we are a walking reaction to what has been encoded in the collective consciousness. The way to affect this is through prayer and meditation, which neutralizes the negative input of the media, society, education, and childhood. It is in these contemplative moments that all the information begins to be re-qualified and starts to be cleansed.

According to Reverend Michael, there are as many forms of meditation as there are people. "The technique is not what is important. Although some teachers may disagree with that and think technique is important, my feeling is that with earnestness and sincerity any technique that your heart loves will be transformational. If you have a desire to grow spiritually, to see the face of God, to know your oneness with pure spirit, those qualities of mind and being will make whatever technique you use magnificent. You can watch the breath in meditation, do a mantra or breathing exercises, contemplative meditation, read scripture or poetry or something that feeds your soul. No matter what you do, with sincerity and earnestness comes transformation."

Some people have the fantasy that they are going to sit down and meditate and it will be so quiet that they will hear a small voice . . . and after two or three sittings they will be instantly enlightened.

This rarely happens, but by embracing the difficulty of the meditation process a student can actually move forward in his practice. Reverend Michael uses the metaphor of a washing machine to explain the process. He says, "That chatter and incessant talking inside your head is all part of the refining, cleansing, and releasing process. It is what I call the agitation cycle in a washing machine. We put in the dirty clothes and a little soap powder, then turn on the machine. At some point, the machine starts to agitate. You can't skip that cycle or you won't have clean clothes. You can't just skip to spin dry where everything is smooth. There has to be agitation to actually clean the dirt out." And when someone feels agitated while meditating, it's actually something being released. He adds, "There are moments in meditation where you have a brilliant insight, a revelation, a healing, or perhaps forgiveness. You see things differently and begin to live from that new level. But then the process begins again. You agitate some more stuff, spin it dry, and then have an insight. You pass through the different stages and move to the other side, which is joyful. Then you begin to understand the process. After a while, you can hold it all in joy, even when you are in pain."

Prayer is similar to meditation in its effects upon the body. There is a saying in twelve-step programs that meditation is listening to God and prayer is talking to God. The power of prayer has been much documented over the years. People all over the world have recovered from devastating illnesses after mass prayers have been conducted.

There is a woman in Hawaii known as Auntie Momie, a Hawaiian Kahuna who carries on her family legacy of Ho'oponopono, which is about forgiveness and the gift and power of prayers. After falling down a flight of stairs and becoming paralyzed, Auntie Momie realized that her accident happened in order to bring her to her life's calling of praying with people and healing them. People from all over the world go to Auntie Momie's home for prayer.

Auntie Hattie Domingo is the last person in her family to practice Ho'oponopono. She explains that Ho'oponopono means to make everything about your life in alignment and right with God. She says, "You may not call it God, you may call it the Creator, Great Spirit, Supreme Being, Jehovah, but there is only one Creator over this whole universe, and this earth. People can make things right by changing their behavior. Ho'oponopono is about forgiveness. Hawaiians say, 'Nothing ever goes right unless you ask for forgiveness. And are able to give forgiveness.'"

The Hawaiians believe that your spirit can leave your body when having a traumatic incident such as an accident or an illness. When this happens, a kahuna is called to call back your spirit. *Uhane* means "spirit," and *hele* means "going," thus the prayer is called the *Uhane Hele.* The interpretation of this Hawaiian prayer for calling the *uhane* back is: "Oh, God, who created the heavens and the earth, and all living things, therein, please return the spirit of _____," and you name the person. "Put it back in his or her body. Don't let it wander from here and there, from house to house, on this earth." When people come to her for prayers, she always asks them to look at the good side and not dwell in the negative. She believes that if one thinks good thoughts, then good thoughts come back to that person.

She also tells them to learn to open their hearts, accept, and love no matter what.

Although in the end my mother was not able to heal her body, her mind, emotions, and spirit healed in a most remarkable way. I learned that how long a person lives is not as important as the quality of life they have. Surprisingly, I also learned that the actual experience of dying can also be greatly healing. A great gift that came from this healing journey with my mother was the discovery of a multitude of alternative and ancient healers and healing modalities. Each healing way integrates the mind, body, and spirit connection and in this way assists in creating wholeness and well-being in a person.

Butch Artichoker, a contemporary Lakota healer who uses his hands in healing, as well as ceremony, herbs, and regressive hypnosis, firmly believes that there is a difference between healing and curing and that sometimes healing is more important even though a person's life may not be saved. He shares, "The spiritual and the mental and the emotional part of the healing are so much more important for the person, even if they have to leave. The importance of looking at what brought all of this on is just as important as the effect of curing. Many healers have the capacity to heal almost any illness there is. I've seen that before, where my wife and I have done a healing for someone with cancer or another serious disease, and the cancer clears up completely within a very short time, so you know that the potential, the healing capacity is there. And then when you work with another person and do a healing very little may happen. The difference is that one person wants to deal with the emotional cause of the illness and the other person is afraid to deal with the emotional cause. I've learned over a long period of time that when it comes to healing, there is an emotional basis to the illness or to the condition. And when people fail to look into and try to heal the emotional cause, it is very difficult to heal the effect, the physical condition."

Butch and his wife, Billie, have worked with people with health challenges such as bulimia, anorexia, and a lot of abuse cases, whether it be physical, emotional, or sexual abuse. He says that there is a very high percentage of people who have these challenges. "We have also worked with people who've had cancer, using hypnosis as a means of looking into that. Sometimes people don't go far enough looking into the causes, and because there's too much there to look at, they won't go too much further. But some people will stick with it and benefit greatly. So we use hypnosis and look at the causes and heal the incidents where these causes lie, and then we bring in the other elements of healing."

He remembers having a patient who was a bright young woman, almost twenty years old, who had a chronic condition of precancerous dysplasia. They worked on her with hypnosis and could see causes and layers of causes. Since there was a time element involved they used plant medicine, a sweat lodge prayer, energy healing, and hypnosis—four different pieces all put together to help her heal. He remembers, "The doctors wanted to operate. As we went along, of course she had examinations done, Pap smears and pelvic exams. The very initial condition was cleared immediately but then the dysplasia of course they could tell by blood tests. And it kept getting better and better as we went along, and then finally disappeared altogether after that, over about a six-and-a-half-month period."

Butch believes that the person's subconscious really knows where the problems lie, so the subconscious goes to where the big problems are. He explains, "If you have a self-worth problem, I don't need to sit and talk with you for a long period of time to find out what caused that self-worth problem. You're going to have some thoughts about it yourself, in terms of where it came from. But if we go into a session and I tell your subconscious I want you to go to an important cause of that, you may go to something you never realized was there. That's when the positive aspect of the healing begins to affect the person, because if you've lost a sense of self at age twelve and we're able to bring that sense of self back, you're going to have a lot more substance to your own emotional well-being than you had before the work."

Butch's own healing crisis with depression brought him to the traditional healers of his tribe during the mid-seventies. He shares, "I went through a very strong depression, and I felt a certain hostility toward Western methods of healing for this type of thing. So I turned to our own healers. And in turning to our own healers, of course it had to practice within the traditional framework, and it reinforced my interest and enthusiasm for learning about spirituality and metaphysics."

During his period of reconnection Butch unexpectedly started having dreams and visions and experiences that at first he did not understand. He shares, "I got a lot of help from Elmer Running with interpretation. I would have many of these dreams and visions interpreted on a fairly regular basis. And that helped me a lot."

Part of Butch's early visions and dreams contained an image of fire coming out of his hands. At first he said he didn't understand the meaning. Then he says, "I began to realize that I have this gift in my hands, and I was ready to use it. And within a matter of forty-eight hours or so, I was beginning to get requests, not just from my family but from outside the family, from people to attempt to cure or heal some problem that they had, and so I began to use my hands more and more. And my wife Billie was very interested in trying to use her abilities as well. So we began to work together, doing healing with our hands and other things such as eagle feathers and eagle fans. Energy can be passed not only through your hands, but it can be passed through objects as well. That is part of our way."

Butch enjoys working with his wife Billie doing healings because, "I feel that I'm the male and the masculinity passes through me and she's female and feminine energy passes through her, and this creates a balance. So we can work as a team in that kind of healing."

Butch would like to see more acceptance for spiritual technology in the medical establishment. He says, "I think too that it would be very helpful for medical schools to bring known healers in, to create some sort of bridge of discussion. Because when I'm doing healing for someone, my concern is about that patient, it's not about whether I'm the one responsible for the healing. It doesn't matter who's responsible for the healing; it's really more important to see the person getting results from both styles, both techniques. We don't have to be in opposition to one another. We're made up of body, mind, and spirit, and if we're only treating the body and the mind, we're not getting far enough."

Butch uses plants as part of his healing technique, and today homeopathy—a natural science that uses various plants, minerals, or animals in very small doses to stimulate the sick person's natural defenses—is used by many people in the United States. Butch says, "Plants have been used by all cultures all over the world for thousands of years and they are very effective. I think one of the things about plants is that you become more and more aware of your own spirituality, you recognize that they're like people too. You know, they have nations and some of them can harm, some of them can heal us. And you establish a relationship with these plants, and you acknowledge them as though they're a person. You know, you ask their permission, you ask them to do this work for the people, because they're here for that purpose. They're here to provide us with oxygen, they're here to provide us with various chemicals that they are able to store, but they have qualities beyond that too. You can use them on their own, and in some cases I do that, but when you use them in conjunction with another they're very potent."

Jana Shiloh, cofounder of the Pacific Academy of Homeopathic Medicine in California, understands the importance of creating and maintaining balance in the mental, emotional, physical, and spiritual body, and of using a noninvasive treatment to obtain this. She became aware of homeopathy during a particularly difficult time in her life and saw a homeopathic practitioner who gave her remedies that helped to create balance and harmony in her life. She shares, "I was going through a divorce, and I was in an emotional as well as a spiritual crisis. I hadn't been able to sleep and would be up at night crying and pacing. After I took the remedies, it all stopped. I then began having glimmers of joy in my life. I was so amazed that there was something that could release me from this state that I felt had me in its grip, that I felt that I had to learn more about homeopathy. When I returned two weeks later to see the practitioner, before I even told him how much better I was feeling, he asked me if I would like to work for him part-time for a few months."

Jana explains that the idea in homeopathy is that we trust that the body has its own natural intelligence and that it can heal itself. However it will often get stuck in its own patterns and not be able to move into healing mode. She says, "What we do in homeopathy is to find substances that have been known to actually create the same symptoms in a so-called healthy person as we see in someone who's out of balance. And in giving minute amounts of this substance, or even energetic amounts to an individual, it has been known to create the same pattern of symptoms. It actually stimulates the body into healing itself. So basically what we're looking for is for the individual to be able to heal himself or herself with a little external stimulation. The remedies are all made from natural substances—animal, mineral, plant kingdoms—and they have been diluted and tapped many times till there's nothing left of the original substance but the energetic healing pattern, or a hologram of that substance."

Homeopathy helps to balance whatever is out of balance. Jana says, "There's no way that we can kill bacteria with homeopathy, but we can stimulate the body to a point where it's not susceptible to that bacteria or virus. Homeopathy really can work on all levels. We have incredible remedies for injury and trauma, and that's something that everyone can learn. For example, most of the time there's one remedy that's used for swelling and bruising, called arnica. It's great for pre- and postoperative conditions, and it actually reduces the healing time and reduces pain after surgery because when you can keep the swelling down, you keep the pain down." Arnica is sold in health food stores, but the highest potencies are obtained from practitioners.

Jana describes the case of a child who had fallen off of a horse. His spleen was over two-thirds mangled. She says, "When the child was in the hospital, they did a CAT scan and said that his spleen could not be saved, that they were going to have to remove it in the morning. His mother had taken a class in homeopathy, and she talked to the doctor and asked if she could give him a homeopathic remedy. He said, 'yeah, go ahead.' She gave him arnica all night long, and by the morning they were amazed to see that his spleen was starting to heal. They were very skeptical, but they decided to wait another eight hours. And eight hours later his spleen was doing even better. And in the end, this eight-year-old child did not have to lose his spleen."

Similar to Jana, Dr. Roy Nakai, dentist and medical intuitive, turned to alternative healing modalities during his own healing crisis with gouty arthritis when he was thirty-nine. He did not want to undergo the normal conventional prednisone and gout treatments for this condition. He explains, "I went on the Melvin Page diet, and during two and a half years I got rid of all of the acid crystals in my system and have been symptom free ever since."

Roy says that "people get sick because there is usually an imbalance that has occurred in the system due to emotional, physical, environmental, inherited, or spiritual reasons. People get better when they become aware of the imbalances that may be contributing to their dysfunction or disease. They need to re-create balance. People can be open to the healing that comes from a Higher Power, depending on their spiritual beliefs. They just have to understand that there are forces and energies outside of their physical being that can assist them in re-creating balance and healing."

Roy has worked with many kinds of people with differing health challenges. "Alternative therapy relies so much on the patient's willingness to make changes, and that is where the difficulty lies both in the results and assessment."

As a dentist Roy has learned about the role of the mouth and teeth in relationship to overall health. "Teeth are an interwoven part of the body that have an effect on the overall health and have a tremendous impact on a patient's overall health and balance. These imbalances must be addressed as part of the total system. Similarly, there is an increasing concern about the effect of some dental filling material on the health of the whole body."

Like Roy Nakai, Margaret Ayers is on the forefront of alternative therapies. Margaret was the first to publish research on utilizing EEG neurofeedback to treat head trauma, stroke, and quadriplegia. Her pioneering neurofeedback equipment design and innovative work have won her international recognition. For twenty years, Margaret has been providing EEG neurofeedback training to clients from all over the world.

Current brain research has shown that neurofeedback can be an effective adjunct to the treatment of brain disorders, head injury, coma, stroke, autism, epilepsy, migraine cluster headaches, attention deficit disorder, dyslexia, learning disabilities, clinical depression, Parkinson's, and post-viral damage.

"We are now able to see the brain waves in less than a thousandth of a second," Margaret says, "between when they occur in the brain and when you see them on the screen. And because we can actually see the brain waves that fast, it allows us to treat problems and health issues that we could never treat before. For example, before we could not treat open head injury, we could not bring people out of deep comas, we could not treat strokes. These people were told to go home, drink tea, and nothing could be done. But now we can go directly to the brain on the motor cortex, or sensory cortex, and train specific areas of the brain to function. We can go to the leg area of the brain. We can go to the arm area of the brain. We could not do that with biofeedback before."

Neurofeedback helps to improve functions such as concentration, short-term memory, speech, motor skills, sleep, energy level, and emotional balance. Margaret says that "the results of the training are permanent unless another trauma or injury occurs. Once the brain's normal rhythmic patterns have been restored, the neurofeedback training is no longer necessary. The effect of neurofeedback training is similar to the effect of training wheels on a bicycle. Once you learn to balance by yourself, the training wheels are no longer needed. The body does not forget."

Through my mother's and my healing journey, I explored universal truths of healing that can be found in the Western culture of modern medicine as well as in the ancient and alternative modalities of healing. It became clear to me that in life there are infinite possibilities available to us all. Larry Dossey talks about the future of the "New Medicine" that will not only include our thoughts and emotions, but will also have a place for something that we have yet to take more seriously—the spiritual dimension of health. Larry recognizes that "spirituality and consciousness are the basic starting point for everything else. Almost all wisdom traditions, almost all esoteric expressions of the great religions honor this perspective, that the fundamental ground of all being is spirit and one of the ways of expressing this is that we must live our life from the inside out—beginning with this understanding."

Chapter Six

"I believe an artist works with the pain. It's our work to see beyond the pain."
—Rickie Byars-Beckwith

"You can't write" was the recurring message I received from most of my teachers in high school. Ten years later, I sat on the edge of the bed in agony, feeling alone and not knowing how to move through the pain of my divorce and the accumulated hurt I had repressed for most of my twenty-eight years. I felt a strong urge to write down my feelings, and yet I held myself back—still harboring a sense of shame about my writing. For many years I buried any desire to express myself through writing.

The pain pushed me to reevaluate what was important to me. Was it more important what other people thought about me or how I felt about myself? In a few moments I was thinking, "The heck with grammar and punctuation. I need to express myself and to purge myself of this pain. The only person I need to be clear for is myself. It doesn't matter what anyone else thinks about what I write, because I am writing for myself and that is enough. I am enough." I was determined to heal and transform the pain that was keeping me from experiencing joy in my life.

As I picked up the pen, I felt a heavy weight lifting. I chose to write from my heart, for myself, without allowing a critic to partake in this sacred ritual. And in doing so, I began the journey of rediscovering my creative self.

In writing I joined together once again with the many parts of who I am that I had lost touch with. I was so accustomed to seeing myself as others perceived me, but now I was getting to know myself from the inside out. My perceptions were shifting, and as I cleared the top layers of hurt and pain I began to gain a greater insight into the deeper meaning behind many life experiences. I was beginning to feel a newfound love for myself and for life.

I discovered that our creative selves are not only about partaking in the arts but also about how well we live our lives and use our creativity to find solutions to life's challenges. In truth, how well we create determines how well our lives work. When we are in pain we are taught to close our hearts and minds and to retreat, to clam up. Retreat has become an unconscious response to pain, yet in reality we discover possibilities for bringing peace and joy into our lives by becoming aware of the creative beings that we are. When our jobs, our marriages, our friendships become painful, we lose touch with how to recognize and express our feelings in a way that will not hurt ourselves nor anyone else. We push the feelings down. The truth is that from this closed place there is no room for creating possibilities for healing and transformation. Our lives will continue to be painful unless we create a pathway for love and healing to move through.

I discovered this most vividly one day while writing this book. I noticed for a couple of days that I was becoming overwhelmed with all the interviews, writing, bills to be paid, and balancing mothering with the rest of my commitments and passions. I had not been to ballet class in nearly a week and I was feeling the loss of not integrating my body, mind, and spirit with the music and movement that nourish my soul. Leaping, turning, adagio are part of who I am and how I connect to myself and other dancers with spirit. I felt sad because I was too tired and had too many commitments to go to dance class. I had promised myself that I would not let go of ballet like I had in the past when other responsibilities took priority. I realized that my health and well-being suffered by letting go of something I felt such a passion for, so missing a class again was painful.

I decided to first get some sleep, because that was the most loving thing I could do for myself. Rather than run myself ragged like I had in the past, I decided I would take time to give myself my own dance class and reawaken my higher feelings that had become ordinary and painful. I turned on music from "The Secret Garden," because it always evokes deep feelings that I tend to bury or ignore. I also love to move to this music.

I became aware that the pain I was feeling was the pain of not being true to my passionate self. Through stretching my body, opening my heart, and allowing my spirit to soar I was able to remember, feel, and become the beauty, love, passion, and peace that I was so longing for. I realized that when we don't use what we have it is painful. I knew that the way to my feeling joy again was to open my heart.

Best-selling author Iyanla Vanzant also had her creativity stifled as a young woman. She says, "When I was a child, nobody ever paid attention to my papers or helped me with my homework, so I felt I didn't matter, that my work didn't matter." But she too wrote for herself and explains, "My writing has not been for anybody. It has been a way for me to express what I was feeling and not allowing myself to feel. All my writing started with journaling, and I never sat down to write a book—ever. I'm writing this for myself, and if others get helped in the process that's good. But trust me, this is not about saving you—this is about saving myself." For Iyanla, having the understanding of how to move into that creative place within herself to help ease the pain, face it, feel it, and ultimately transform it has been of paramount importance in her life.

In Iyanla's book *The Spirit of Man*, the healing was around her father and becoming aware of how this relationship manifested itself into all others in her life. And she was angry. She shares, "In writing the book and listening to what was being said to me, I learned to listen from my heart, not my brain. I don't hear it and debate and think about it; I hear it and it resonates through my body and then it just breaks down everything else. I can have no resistance to it. I don't know if it's true or not true, I don't even care. I know when it comes like that I have to put it down. There is another energy moving through me with my own energy, and it's a whole different kind of level, and the more it is done the more I can maintain it a little longer each time."

Jack Canfield, coauthor of the best-selling book *Chicken Soup for the Soul,* a self-esteem expert, and a therapist, also discovered that reconnecting with his creative self is a deep process. Jack believes that for him there are two sources of creativity. One is his own experience. And then there's also a higher source, which he describes as coming from his higher self. "I think if you're overly involved in your emotions, then you're not in touch with your higher self, and that certainly can cut off the flow of that aspect of creativity."

Jack is most in alignment with a model of psychology called psychosynthesis, which basically says we have a higher self that is the source of our greatest creativity and the highest qualities such as love and compassion. It's the place where poets like Rumi write from. Other psychological functions are more into the personality level, such as our minds, our emotions, our imaginations, our physical sensory selves, our bodies, something we call "desire," and then intuition.

He believes that everyone has had writer's block, and everyone has had times when there is no inspiration. He also believes there are tools to use to reconnect. "There are books about how to get through writer's block, how to close your eyes and get in touch with your inner muses, and those kind of activities are certainly useful."

But today, Jack focuses more on learning to go with his natural rhythms. He realizes the importance of being centered so you can receive the inspiration for your creativity. "When you look at Nature as a metaphor, you can't give birth 365 days a year. It's just not possible. No animal could do that. There's a period of getting pregnant, there's a period of dormancy, there's a period of growth, then there's a period where the thing in you just has to come out. And you would be fighting yourself to keep it in. The contractions are just happening. And I get periods where I just write and write and write and write, and if anyone interrupts me it's 'leave me alone.' It's kind of the way an animal focuses on giving birth and just shuts out the rest of reality.

"And then once you've given birth, you have to take care of that which you've birthed. It's a different process. Right now, I'm writing a book called *The Success Principle,* so I'm spending a couple of hours every morning on it. And I write until I feel like I don't want to write anymore. And I used to plan my writing and say 'I will do two hours on this.' I would sit there no matter what telling myself, 'I will get this done,' and I would push through my resistance. But I'm seeing now that that's like saying I'm going to inhale for two hours. I mean, your lungs would burst. You can't do it. So now much more than before, if I'm writing, and I don't want to do it, I get up, take a walk, go do something else, and wait until I feel like sitting down again."

It's important to recognize that we should honor our natural rhythms when we're engaged in a creative endeavor. Pushing "through the resistance," as Jack says, rarely accomplishes anything. And being in touch with our higher self or spiritual self is often necessary. Stephen Simon, producer of the movie *What Dreams May Come* and cofounder of the film production company called Metafilmics, spent years feeling ostracized, criticized, and laughed at in the film business. That was during the 1980s, when he could not get *What Dreams May Come* off the ground for many years. He explains, "All the doors were closed for me. I thought to myself, 'OK,

I'm wrong. This isn't going to happen and I have to move on.' Rather than trying to figure out another way to do it, I just said, 'OK, I can't do this.' I took all of the creative aspects that I felt about this entire area and repressed them. I went through a very rough time until I finally got onto a spiritual path and consciously came back to myself. Even when I was succeeding with certain projects, I never really felt a part of the film business because I just couldn't get into the mind-set. It took me coming into my spirituality to realize that there is nothing wrong with the mind-set of the industry the way it is, nor is there anything wrong with the fact that I'm not comfortable being a part of it. So it was really a question of accepting myself."

BUT what happens when your creative gift is interrupted by an accident? For Alaine Haubert, former principal ballerina for the Joffrey Ballet and American Ballet Theatre, the journey of rediscovering her creative self was excruciatingly painful. During a rehearsal, Haubert was dropped by her dance partner and severely injured. She was told that she would never walk again, and her back injury caused enormous pain.

She says, "But the psychological and emotional pain went far beyond that. That was the pain that no one else could really perceive. I had identified completely with being a ballet dancer, and that was my safety place. Now what was I going to do?" Alaine was just thirty-two years old and felt that her life was completely over.

"I was lying in the hospital in traction on Demerol, and traction means you can't move. I felt like a butterfly, a live butterfly, stuck with a pin through its heart. That was the pain and the image that kept coming to me. I was there for three weeks. And the people I had been dancing with for ten years in the Joffrey Ballet had gone away to do a film for PBS, and no one was around, including my husband. And the people who I thought were my friends, my peers, my colleagues, were so involved in what they were doing, including my husband, that no one called me while I was in the hospital, going through the worst pain of my life."

As she lay in the hospital and looked at her future, she accepted that she would never dance again. But she also realized that she didn't want to continue with the life she had created up to that point, because she couldn't handle it without dance. Dance had helped her escape. That meant leaving a marriage that was no longer working and creating a new life. Alaine says, "The journey within has not always been straight, as no journey is. It has had many curves, many adventures, and lots of lessons. But I quickly got that I was here for a purpose, and I knew that it would be a very good idea to figure out what that was, as fast as possible."

Alaine started to use visualization techniques to help her heal, and she believes this was a turning point in her recovery. She says, "I started to visualize what my body looked like without the muscles. I went into the bones and nerves. I took a journey inside of myself, I found my lower back, I found where the nerve damage was. I somehow took a trip inside of myself—I figured out where the real injury was, exactly what had happened, and I thought, you know what, if I keep dwelling on that spot, I'm never going to get well! That's when I started thinking about rotating my ankles, doing a little neck stretch, pointing and flexing my feet—I'm a ballet dancer, I've been dancing since I'm five. I thought, well, I could do some stretches maybe that don't affect my back—started doing a little breathing, and that was the day I started getting well. It took a long time, months and months and rehabilitation."

Alaine realized that in order to support herself she would have to teach ballet. It gave her a great deal of pleasure, and she found out it was another arena for her to perform in. She remembers, "There were many ways I could use my magic, my gifts, that I had no idea were possible. So I learned as I taught. The more I taught, the more I learned. And I've been teaching now for some twenty-five years." To Alaine's surprise she was contacted by Kevin McKenzie, a dance partner of hers from the Joffrey Ballet, who had since gone on to be principal dancer at American Ballet Theatre. He told her he was planning to take over American Ballet Theatre and asked Alaine if she would be the ballet mistress for the dance company. At the time she was living in Hawaii, but she took the job and moved to New York. Alaine worked there for four years and then moved to California.

Alaine's belief about her purpose in life has shifted dramatically over the years. She says, "Each of us is here for several reasons. I feel that we're here on the one hand to be kind to each other, treat each other as best we can, everybody, and everything. I also feel that we choose to be here to refine ourselves at the level of the soul. And for everybody, that's different. That refining process can take many versions, many paths, many ways, but the ultimate goal is to refine our souls into a point of vibration, beauty, and clarity."

Alaine Haubert's story is touching because of the graceful way she has found her life's work. Her creative expression of dance took on new meaning when she found herself unable to perform as a principal dancer. But she went within and sought deeper meaning to how she could express herself differently. If faced with an obstacle that blocks our creative outlet, there may be other ways.

Iyanla Vanzant knows she is not alone in her endeavors and that allows her the freedom to let anything happen. She says, "The creativity is co-creation with God, and if you're doing what God tells you to do, you're going to be creating something for God's purpose. For me, it's writing, for you, it may be dancing. If you just develop a partnership with the God self, with God, you will be creating, if nothing else, a new idea, and everything is an idea. Then you develop the strength and courage to act on that idea and that's what puts shape and form and matter to the idea and makes it a thing. And anything that God creates is good so somebody is going to be helped or healed by it. I believe the whole creativity is just developing the partnership with God, that's what heals the pain because it's not you anymore."

Like Alaine, novelist Isabel Allende journeyed to the underworld after experiencing devastating pain and triumphantly returned with renewed wisdom, courage, and compassion. Isabel has an interesting point of view regarding her writing—she believes that she couldn't have been a writer at a young age. She says, "I would have not been a writer at twenty, because I needed forty years of my life, of struggle, to get to the point where I could be a writer. I couldn't be a writer before. But all the creative force was there, repressed. Waiting for an opportunity to manifest itself."

One of her most poignant struggles was when her daughter, Paula, fell into a coma and eventually died. Isabel began writing at Paula's bedside to help deal with the fear and pain. Isabel says, "For the whole year, I wrote all the basis of what was the book *Paula*. So creating the book pulled me out of the pain." But after finishing the book, she fell into a depression and couldn't write for three years. Eventually, Isabel found the courage to write again, and she has confidence now that she will always write. Her writing, she says, is a gift to help her transform her pain. She elaborates, "I think that I moved through the different forms of pain writing. Writing is what has allowed me to move. And what is the writing? The writing is not the material thing of putting words on a piece of paper. It is the hours you spend alone. It's a journey inside, inside yourself to start with. And even if you're creating fiction, you're creating something that has nothing to do with your own life. It's the time you spend alone in silence listening to voices, to stories that I think are there in the air."

The process of creativity is intuitive to Isabel. She says, "I'm like a radio, and I will be trying this little knob back and forth until I catch the wave. And I will hear the voices. I have to relax. It's like sex. If you are thinking of what you have to do, or following the manual, it doesn't work! It only works when you surrender to the process. And I think that the creativity comes from that, from self-confidence that the process will carry you."

Moving through pain into transformation and rebirth, Isabel most eloquently shares her journey from the depths of her soul. She offers a greater understanding of how tragedy and loss can act as a catalyst for creating in us greater wisdom, strength, and love.

Rickie Byars-Beckwith has moved through many layers of the soul in search of her creative self. Rickie is a greatly loved musician, artist, and the director of Agape International Choir. Rickie shares, "Many years ago, my daughter Georgia lay in the hospital bed, unable to see or talk because the tissue in her brain had suddenly begun to swell, and the doctors said she probably would never see again. It was the dark night of my soul. I needed a stronger foundation. I didn't know how to connect with God. The whole ordeal just showed me, in no uncertain terms, that I needed to stand on solid ground and that I needed to get myself together and strengthen my faith."

Rickie recalls how she moved from trying to control situations to understanding that the creative person is about letting go and seeing what needs to be seen. She says, "My language would be, 'God is revealing a Higher order in my life right now.' And that is a co-creation, because you are working with God, 'cause you are taking responsibility. You are working with the Power. I didn't quite understand co-creation then like I do now. Co-creation felt to me like a partnering and partnering felt like there are two not one. And now I know there is only God, and It is in everybody. When I am in my joy, I am an instrument for God. So we work together. But it is such an osmosis path that I don't know where I begin and end; there is no separation. It is more than I can understand."

Rickie further shares, "I believe that an artist works with the pain. It's our work to see beyond the pain and to see the larger picture. For me, sometimes the pain is just the wake-up call to go to the piano. And for other people who aren't musicians, if they can just stop and breathe and remember that they can pray or consciously reach for something inspirational to connect to once again."

Rediscovering our creative self is a most sacred part of the journey toward healing. We each have been blessed with unique gifts that are meant to be expressed and shared. But sometimes it just takes listening to our innermost self and honoring what we hear. Our creative self is our deepest self. And it is not only about partaking in the arts, but it is how well we live our lives and use our creativity to live in harmony with our truths. When we live our life from a closed place, there isn't much room for creating. Healing and transformation occur when we are open to expressing our gifts, whether that be writing, painting, dancing, or whatever we desire to do. And to restore the creative self, one doesn't have to be an artist. Creativity resides in us all and as each person in this chapter says, it's about accessing something within ourselves.

Chapter Seven

"The essence of the universe is always around us, always speaking to us, and it doesn't matter what situation we are in. Death is only a walk through a door into another dimension."
—*Kahu O Te Range*

Mom lay frail, her bones brittle and her body weighing less than eighty pounds. I carefully stroked her in a tentative manner, doing my best to help ease the pain. In a weakened voice, she kept saying, "I'm going to live, aren't I?" I wanted to be fully present and supportive, yet a part of me closed up and felt numb. I told her she would be fine, trying desperately to believe my own words as I continued to comfort her the best I could. As her spirit drifted, so did mine.

In my mother's last days, neither my brother, David, my sister, Michele, nor myself could talk about death. We were not able to tell her how much we would miss her and what a profound loss we each would feel without her. We kept hanging on to the possibility that she would somehow live. We moved from having tremendous hope to living in denial, and as a result we lost the opportunity to assist her in making her transition and to share our last words together from the depths of our souls. Even more painful was the fact that we each separately experienced her loss rather than pulling together and sharing our pain. We were afraid to be vulnerable and authentic with one another. In our upbringing we were not given an understanding of the natural cycles of life and death. We were not rooted to the natural world, and in this sense everyone was unable to come to terms with issues of dying. Disassociation in one area of our life showed up in other areas as well, until we were willing to heal and transform the pain of feeling disconnected.

A profound lesson I learned during the passing of my mother was how important it is to be authentic and share all that is in your heart with the ones you love. While I was stroking her arm during her last hours, I could barely feel anything. I wanted to tell her how much I was going to miss her if she died and how much I loved her, yet I was afraid I would break down and sob uncontrollably and burden her. My fear kept me from showing her all my love in her time of need. She and I shared our love on so many occasions, yet this was the most fitting. I also could not bring myself to tell her good-bye and to talk about her leaving. Neither could she, and we lived in denial— each secretly fearing how we would cope with the loss.

Joan Borysenko, best-selling author and practitioner of mind-body medicine, illustrates how even in the last hours of a loved one's major life transformation can take place, both for the person making their transition as well as for their loved one experiencing the loss. Joan and her mother were each able to see themselves as well as each other in a new light before her mother passed on. They were in the elevator in the hospital when Joan's mother asked her for forgiveness. Joan replied, "Boy, I've made a lot of mistakes too, Mom. There have been so many times that I've judged you, that I haven't been there for you, and I'm sorry and I want to be forgiven too." And that was all it took, fifteen seconds.

"And then we had an interesting little thing happen," Joan says. "I pushed my luck. I said, 'I'd like to exchange a quality with you. Something in your being, in your soul I really admire. You've got courage, and I'm a wimp and I'd like your courage.' And she said, 'You can have it.' And then she said, 'From you, I'd like your compassion.' And that blew me away because I always thought that I had never even shown my own mother any compassion. The fact that she could even see it in me was such an incredible acknowledgment. So we did that. She said good-bye to everybody and then she fell into the last morphine-assisted sleep, at around midnight."

After my mother made her transition, I made the conscious decision that no one would ever understand my pain and that I would have to wade through my sorrow alone. I felt very estranged from my brother and sister, and it seemed that all of the most unhealthy patterns in our family were coming up for healing. There was a lot of judgment of one another and a great sense of separation. I did not have the tools and the understanding of how to be vulnerable with the ones I cherish and love. I also did not know how to fully grieve and move through the mourning period of a loved one with the understanding that death is a natural part of the cycle of life.

In Joan's case, she bonded with her son as the result of being open and vulnerable. At one point as she and her twenty-year-old son, Justin, were keeping vigil by her mother's bedside, Joan had a vision that allowed her to see the clear and pure relationship between mother and child. She remembers, "These kinds of revelations about the perfection of my life with my mother, about how we had learned from one another and the complete circularity of it, of her giving me birth physically and then my giving her soul birth again to the other side, and my being reborn in the process. And when I opened my eyes from this, I saw that everything is made of light, nothing has form anymore, everything is light. And I see that my mother's dead body is made of light."

Joan was given the gift of being able to share this experience with Justin and to create a more honest and authentic parent-child relationship. They both grew in understanding the multidimensionality of our human experience. Joan shares, "It became clear to me that everything is just densities in the light and everything is inter-penetrating and you can see everything is interdependent, everything in the universe is interdependent. And then I looked across my mother's dead body and there was my son, who is literally illuminated. He's made of light with a halo of light and he's weeping tears of great joy. He's awestruck, this look on his face, and he looks at me and says, 'Mom, the room is filled with light, can you see it?' And I told him I could. And he moved over close to me and we sat together with our arms around each other and he said, 'That's Grandma Lilly's last gift.

She's holding open the door to eternity so that we can have a glimpse. You must be very grateful to your mother.' And I said, 'Until this moment I had no gratitude at all. I was really an ingrate. Now I have true gratitude.' And he said, 'She gave you the greatest gift any human being could give another, she gave you her life. She had all this great wisdom and chose not to be able to show it in this lifetime for you.' That was pretty amazing and it was a great teaching in forgiveness."

Joan then asked Justin to forgive her, and she realized how wonderful it was that they could share this way while he was so young. It also took away her fear of death. Joan was able to understand that forgiveness is about nonjudgment. "When I think of how many times I judged my mother, how many times I'm sitting as a psychologist saying this is a person with no insight, she doesn't want to have any insight . . . what a lack of humility, what arrogance I found in myself. Some of that was stripped away. And what I'm convinced of is that in the end only love matters. And that's the important thing. And so in a way, I think death guides my life, because I feel what I really have to do is to live my life with kindness and love."

But what do we do with the pain that won't go away? Or how do we get to a place of willingness to start to heal? After my mother passed, I was haunted by the memories and feelings of her dying from cancer. Witnessing the loss of her life force for two years— from when she appeared to be a healthy woman of 130 pounds who ran four miles three times a week, practiced yoga, and watched her diet, into a woman who required diapers and who weighed almost half her normal weight during her last days—was both devastating and horrifying. I was left feeling powerless, sad, full of fear, and anger. And these feelings seemed to permeate into almost all aspects of my life, leaving me out of balance and in more pain.

Goldie Hawn shares that when her mother died she too felt hopeless. She says, "It was as if I had no one else to dance for. She was the one that I was dancing for. She was the one who I was being what I am for, because I wanted to please my mother. I wanted her to be proud. I took pride in that. And when that was taken away, I didn't even know why I was doing what I was doing. I questioned why I was in show business. What's the use? Because nobody else really cares, not that way."

But, we have to learn to move forward. Rigoberta Menchú Tum taught me many great lessons as she went through the horrific experience of having her family, friends, and community die in a brutal and violent manner during the political unrest in Guatemala in the late seventies and early eighties. Rigoberta found healing in giving and sharing. "I believe nothing can be greater than the love people have for each other. For ten years after the death of my parents, I thought I would live my life as a wanderer, a permanent traveler. During those ten years I was asked in many interviews whether I would ever marry. 'What for,' I would say, 'when I have the opportunity to support three children's nurseries.' There were three children's nurseries where I would go occasionally to visit 'my children.' I would take them toys I had collected from wherever I had been. There was another nursery in Nicaragua, so we had established two nurseries where we could save the children, especially those children of Guatemalan comrades who had been murdered. The mothers of the children were working for human rights, so it was important to have a place for them."

Rigoberta found meaning in her pain, but the legacy of violence brought great hardship and calamity to Rigoberta's own family. "My brother Victor was married and had four children. When he was killed two of his children died of malnutrition. They couldn't live. His other two children lived a very, very difficult life."

On her healing path, Rigoberta discovered that "all people who have endured pain have also increased their human and spiritual sensitivity." She shares, "I have been by the side of many people who have suffered pain. I have personally seen things. It seems life has tested me by putting me very close to the most negative things. But I feel that those lives that are extinguished remain with me as a strength, and I have converted it into a weapon of persuasion for others: to be humble, to respect life so they will not abandon those who are most needy, to not take a happy moment for granted, to take good care of their family, to love their children, to feel connected. Finally, I feel many whom I have seen are with me."

In grieving the loss of a loved one, it is natural to feel angry, and even more so when the death is untimely and violent in nature. What we do with that anger and how we heal and transform it is of great importance in the renewal of oneself after the death of a loved one. Rigoberta's anger and pain gave her great understanding of the importance of continuing her parent's work and not allowing their struggles to be in vain. She says, "The anger I felt was not directed toward hunting down those responsible for the death of my mother. Rather it was directed to seeking out the truth. I wanted to imagine coming face-to-face with those responsible, those who had killed, tortured, and raped my mother. I wanted someday to see them face-to-face and I thought that although it would be painful, I would want to be told what had happened to my mother. So my cause became struggling for truth, to know the truth about everyone from the first detail to the last. And of course, my cause became finding my slain family's remains. I felt I had to finish the social struggle they had not yet completed." Rigoberta used her pain to fight against the oppression that she saw happening throughout her country. But, she still had to grieve and feel her feelings.

It is natural to feel afraid after having experienced violence targeted at one's family and people. Yet Rigoberta knew not to let her fear drive her into becoming violent, as her violators had been. Instead, she understood that her power lay within herself, and she used her intuitive abilities to gain understanding and a sense of control in her life. And this gave her hope. She shares, "Many times I was afraid, very afraid. I felt especially fearful that I would never again see my little sister. For twelve years I had only one feeling, that my sister was alive. And then one day my sister Ana appeared with two small children. I felt so much happiness. My sister had named her daughter Maya Rigoberta because she wanted to honor my name. She knew I was alive because my voice would come over the radio and she saw me in the media. She felt very proud of me but was unable to make contact. When the family was reunited it was a great wonder that reinforced my feelings once more to have a family of my own."

As human beings it is natural to want to feel connected to one another. But out of fear and ignorance, we build walls and create separation. When we move through our pain and take down the walls, we
are able to feel connected and supported, which is so necessary when
we need to heal from the loss of a loved one. Rigoberta understands
this and says, "I had many friends who helped me. There were persons who listened many hours to me as I spoke about what had happened to my family, and remembered the good things about my
family."

Rigoberta chooses what she wants to remember and how she
wants to remember her loved ones. "Imagining my dead ones as being alive is very important to me. I also think it gives me a goal to develop my own positive attitude. Because I cannot imagine them dead.
I do not want to imagine my mother being tortured. Rather I want to
imagine her as a normal woman. This means that at any given moment I can ration the pain in that moment, because imagining the
horror is different than imagining the good things about my dear
ones that I lost."

Dreams help to guide us and are a way to stay connected to our
loved ones. For Rigoberta, certain dreams helped her make more direct connections with her deceased family. She shares, "I would dream
my father was fairly happy, and I would dream of him working on
our land. I would dream of him bringing a river for the village. In my
dreams he was very communicative with me. I dreamed of my mother
a few times. Something significant in these dreams with my mother is
that I never had the opportunity to speak with her. I always have

seen her combing or braiding her hair. But there is no real communication, and I almost always know beforehand that that is what I
will dream about. These dream times have helped me to develop my
own positive attitude."

Rigoberta was able to find renewal in knowing that she is dearly
loved. She explains, "In our Maya religion, if one loses their family,
if all is lost, brother, father, mother, it is necessary to look for a new
family. You need to find a new home, a new family. Your age does not
matter. You may be older or younger. But, being an orphan technically does not exist because there is always a new family to love, to
adore. And I found my new family in several homes that I love, in
Guatemala, in Italy, and in Mexico. These families loved me as if I
were part of the family. So, I think a person can find true friends,
friends who will love them, and whom they can love and give love in
a special way."

Here in the United States, our culture doesn't as readily embrace
the Mayan thinking in terms of finding another family, but perhaps
we can learn from their ways. I found it difficult to open up to my
brother and sister after our mother died, but I sought healing in
other communities that would accept me. I turned to Native American ceremony and prayer and sought out a therapist to assist me in
moving through my feelings. I spent a lot of time in nature reconnecting my spirit and soul to the natural elements and remembering
my Creator through these elements. I began to learn and accept more
about the natural cycles of life. I read a lot of metaphysical books, eager to learn more about the invisible world. I found like-minded
people to be with and took the time to pamper myself. I noticed that

I was able to move through this period of my life with more ease than when my father died because I was eating more healthfully, cutting out sugar and foods with preservatives, eating lots of fresh vegetables, and taking vitamin supplements. I felt less stressed after the loss than I did with my father, when I was eating very poorly and not growing as much spiritually.

It is difficult enough to lose one's parents, siblings, relatives, and friends. But to have our newborns in this world for just a short time is ever so challenging. Rigoberta also lost a son, Tsunun, when he was less than a year old. When he died she said, "Son, if you go, leave us your smile so we can have many smiles for the years left for us here on earth. Leave us your dreams, your human talents. Leave us everything because we do not have those things in excess; we are in want of them. I would ask you my son, leave me your courage and your strength. Son, it isn't easy for a mother to think that her newly arrived child has to depart. I would have wanted you to be with me. I would have wanted you to suckle at my breast, that you would have received the best that I have. But, if this is the decision of the gods, the powers that be, and our *nahuales* that you must depart, then I must learn to accept this. And I will think of your positive qualities and your courage and your struggle. And we will do all that is good so we won't betray your energies. You will be with us always."

Rigoberta felt better that she could talk to him, and she says that she continues to feel his presence. She says, "We have a relationship even though he is in another place. My children are my most pro-found accomplishment. Having them is very great and gives hope to our lives."

Rigoberta has experienced the most soul-wrenching pain in her life and yet has remarkably been able to keep her faith in good over evil. She shares, "I believe there is a basic condition and that is to believe in humanity. If one believes in humanity, one struggles for humanity. And if one believes in others, then one struggles for others. What happens is that it is more damaging when others fail you or when you fail others. But humanity is infinite. Humanity and the lives of the planet are infinite."

Like Rigoberta, Isabel Allende lost her child, Paula. "I could only see the pain and the horror of it for years and years," Isabel says. "I wrote the book *Paula* immediately after she died, and the process of writing the book allowed me to get through the awful first year. Just the discipline of sitting down at the typewriter and writing every day for eight hours kept me busy and forced me to get out of bed, to get into my clothes, and to come to my office and work. That kept me going, and after the book was published I really felt a mourning, an emptiness, the total void."

While Isabel's grieving process was different than Rigoberta's, she was able to open and become willing to heal and share her healing with the world. An awakening for Isabel was when she was able to look deeply within herself and discover that she had the ability to recognize what she most needed in order to heal. She says, "First I took Prozac for about three months, I went into therapy, and my family took me to Hawaii for a vacation. Then I said, 'What am I doing, this doesn't make any sense. There's no way that I'm not going to feel the pain. The pain is going to come back even worse, I have to go through this and travel the whole underworld and then emerge at the other end of the tunnel someday, somehow.' And that's how it happened—it took five years but it happened."

Isabel received thousands of letters from all over the world after Paula's death. These letters convey women's fears that they won't be loved in the way that Paula was loved or that they won't have a mother or husband like she had. And of course she receives letters from mothers who fear that the same thing would happen to their children. Isabel says, "This made me realize how much fear we live with. I began to understand that part of the pain comes from fear. If we just accept that life is painful and that pain is unavoidable and that pain is a teacher and that it's OK to be in pain, then we start to lose the fear of pain and pain can become very healing. After five years, I have learned to live with Paula's absence, her physical absence, and relate through the spiritual presence in such a way that I think the fear of losing another child, and the fear of death, is gone, or at least it's less present."

For Isabel today, there is still pain. She shares, "It comes in flashes; it's like post-traumatic syndrome. I can be taking a shower and all of a sudden I have a flash of my daughter in a wheelchair and my daughter in intensive care and I scream. The scream comes from I don't know where—it happens still but it happens less. She's contained now, she's my companion permanently. I talk to her all the time." Isabel stays connected to her daughter in other ways, too. "I have a little altar at home that has two drawers, and inside of them I have part of her ashes, I have her picture, I have her love letters . . .

the last letter she wrote to me. I have all of that there—it's contained. Every day when I start writing I light a candle in front of her altar and another candle next to my computer. I open the doors and she's with me, and then when the day's over I blow out the candle and close the doors and she's contained. The pain is contained. In that way I continue on with the rest of the world."

Understanding the meaning of feeling connected and the deeper layers of life's essence assists us in renewal. For Isabel, moments of true connection with her children and grandchildren were when her grandchildren were born. She says, "Those were extraordinary moments of love when I have been connected to another human being in a most profound way."

Through spirituality, psychological counseling, and energetic healing such as EMDR, field touch, and other energy work including acupuncture and healing touch, I have learned to connect with the root of the pain and to heal and transform it, so I can once again know the joy that lies on the other side of pain. Goldie Hawn, too, immersed herself into many spiritual traditions, seeking renewal and greater connection. To help to heal herself, she says, "I read a lot of interfaith writings, I read a lot of religions, I read a lot of the Kabbala, I didn't study only one spiritual way. I read a cross section of many different faiths and religions. And I took myself out of the mud and into a higher place. And I brought my mother with me." She also remembers not getting a lot of work at the time and believes it was really a gift from God, "because I couldn't have done what I did and worked at the same time. The universe said to me, 'No. You don't get to work anymore. You don't get to do anything but pay attention to your own soul and its growth.' And then through this healing time was the time that I really began to become empowered and understand the depth of my own spiritual life. And I spent long hours reading and by myself in my meditation room, to try to come to grips and understanding with death. And with losing my mother, who was so powerful in my life."

Goldie also learned the importance of releasing our tears in the grieving process. She says, "Tears are healing, and they are healing on a metaphysical level, and they're also healing on a physical level because tears are natural antibiotics. Also, tests have been done and results have been proven that tears strengthen the immune system. As does laughter. They're very closely related. It's the connection you have to your heart center. And if you can open up that heart center and feel tears, then you can open up that heart center and feel joy. If you cannot cry, there is a cap on your level of joy appreciation. So, to be given the permission to feel and to cry is being given the permission to laugh. One feeds the other. Low-level depression lowers the immune system. So sorrow and tears are to be expelled, not to be held.

Kahu O Te Range, Maori Kahuna (Polynesian traditional healer), understands the importance of feeling one's loss and expressing the loss with words and tears. He shares, "We enhance the understanding of pain by encompassing it. So when someone dies, people are encouraged to feel the loss. They are encouraged to express themselves through tears and through words, the real loss. And then in understanding that they have departed, we understand that life goes on forever, and they have bridged to a new space of being, and they in essence are pathfinders for us. So you have to go back to the idea of understanding genealogy. That we are here in this present space and we came from our parents and their parents, and their parents and their parents before them, and we work all the way to the gods, and eventually back to the Creator. Whatever that means, whatever your perception of that might be. But we go all the way back, therefore we—the pain and the suffering and the joy and all of that is something that we all inherit. Anyway, it's a DNA memory. If we only experienced joy and no pain, then life is one-dimensional. So pain is a part of life, pain is part of the process of learning and understanding. We have to view it in a very, very positive sense. That pain is basically a way of bridging. When I say pain is awareness of an understanding, I really mean that."

Kahu perceives this as not only being about living, understanding, and encompassment, but about the ability to transcend all the spaces and the time in this space. He shares, "You might say that you and I are here, experiencing life on a linear time scale. But that linear time scale is only a blink of an eye or the beat of a heartbeat when you compare it to the cyclic, linear, and instantaneous time. So you might say that our ancestors are still with us."

Kahu had an experience over thirty years ago in which he gained a greater understanding of relativity and clear understanding of what death is about and what choices we have. He shares, "I was diving off of Carolina Island, by myself, and I was at about 100 feet down. As I was swimming amongst these giant kelp plants, and all of a sudden the leaves and the kelp weaved around me, I was all entangled in this kelp. Then I went through the process of panic, and I distinctly remember removing or pulling my breathing apparatus from my mouth. Then all of a sudden I became unconscious. I wasn't aware of how much water I had taken in.

"Then I went through this whole genetic recall, everything of this lifetime that had occurred to me, my whole life here. And the experience of other things from other dimensions also flashed through. I would call that 'DNA reassessment.' My DNA was deciding whether or not to pass on or to stay. Just as I finished the DNA recall, a multitude of past lives flashed before me. All of a sudden this great spiral opened up and I started going through the spiral. And when I got to the end of the spiral, it was full of light. And there standing at the end of the light was a person that I perceived to be Christ. And the person said one thing, 'Are you coming, or are you staying?' I was given the choice, and I decided I'm staying. The being said to me, 'Yes. You have lots to do.'

"The next thing, in a blink, I was on the surface, and I felt foolish, I had no water in my lungs, I had not embolized, but at that time there must have been a great amount of adrenaline created, because I ripped the kelp off from around me. But I was free, I had no damage to myself, and in itself that was my own miracle. When I said, Yes, I'd like to stay, what flashed before me was to take this experience and empower others to empower themselves, sharing the understanding that the essence of the universe is always around us and always speaking to us, regardless of the situation we are in. The beauty in the transition for me was that I gained an understanding that death is only a walk through a door into another dimension, and there was beauty in that. Yet I chose to stay, for a higher purpose, one, for my own development, so that I could share this passage and this story. And what grew of all of this are some ideas and shaman-istic practices that empower and help people to understand them-selves and life in a more meaningful manner."

One understanding that became clear for Kahu from this experi-ence is "that people keep punishing themselves because of thoughts that keep coming up. What I have learned is that when the thought comes up, breathe the thought, feel what it feels like within the thought, release the thought, and finally transmute it."

Kahu carries within him the wisdom of his ancestors and the ex-periences of today that have taken him on timeless journeys, gaining the most sacred of teachings. He understands his purpose for being here, and inspires the rest of us to connect more intimately with our own true purposes in life. He gives testimony to the idea that we are connected to life on many dimensions.

Sometimes we have experiences that cannot be proven by science, yet greatly assist us in our healing. One particular example occurred when my daughter, Imani, and I were meeting His Holiness the Dalai Lama briefly after a more lengthy meeting with his head rep-resentative to the United States. As I was walking away from shak-ing His Holiness the Dalai Lama's hand at his hotel and feeling as if I was being bathed in white light, I headed to make a phone call in the hotel lobby. As I was talking, a ten-pound piece of metal hanging from the wall fell from eight feet above the ground onto my daughter's head. She was sitting beneath this fixture cross-legged on the ground and waiting for me. I felt it coming and grabbed her, but I could not stop it from hitting her. She screamed profusely and an ambulance was immediately called. We rushed her to the hospital, and after she was thoroughly checked, she was released. We have both never felt more grateful for her well-being.

On the airplane flying back home to Hawaii, Imani suddenly called to me, "Mom, do you see Grandma Sylvia?" I said no, and then I asked, "What does she look like?" The first thing she said was that she was wearing bright red lipstick. I couldn't believe it. My mother and I fought over her red lipstick almost daily when I was a young girl. I was embarrassed by it because the fire-engine red was too bright for my taste. We did not have any pictures of her in color from that early age, so Imani could not have seen her with that lipstick on. In later years she wore a dark pink lipstick. Imani was so surprised by my mother's appearance outside of the airplane window, looking about forty years old, wearing a blouse and skirt and of course her bright red lipstick, that she accidently knocked over the orange juice she was drinking. She then shared that Grandma said, "I will always be with you, Imani."

Imani told me she felt Grandma was an angel who was sent to watch over her and who helped save her life at the hotel. She then went on to express that she felt Grandma was also responsible for protecting her when she was three years old and had fallen headfirst out of a van window onto a paved driveway. Imani walked away from that fall with a small cut on her chin.

We both felt more rooted and connected after having experienced my mother's presence. I believe that it is also possible to heal these feelings even after our loved ones have made their transition. It is not as important to debate about whether what a person experienced is true or not. If a person feels more rooted and connected as a result of a vision, then healing is taking place.

In our effort to heal and renew ourselves after the death of a loved one, it is common to seek greater understanding about what happens after we die and how can we can continue to feel connected to our loved ones after they have made their transition. Barbara Brennan, energy healer and founder of the Barbara Brennan School of Healing, sees energy and is able to connect with people who have died. She shares, "Often after people die, I see them right away and I can converse with them. So I know there's a continued existence, but there's still great pain in the physical loss." Barbara explains that when people die, they may not look the same as they did when they were alive. She says, "When my father died, he came as he looked. And I had an experience with my friend, Marjorie, who oftentimes looks different, but she is playing a harp. She used to complain toward the end of her life that the harp didn't have enough strings with high notes. Now the harp she plays has more strings on it."

Barbara channels someone called "Heyoan" who explains who he is: "You might call me 'Barbara's oversoul.' You might call me 'the one that Barbara is becoming,' or you might call me 'the one that Barbara is,' depending on which level one looks at, or from what vantage point you see this. I might be called 'Barbara's main guide.' I also share the same core essence with Barbara, and I am one who has finished my rounds of incarnation and yet at the same time I am incarnated at this particular point in Barbara."

Heyoan's perception of death is this: "We could describe death from our vantage point as simply a homecoming, or a birthing into our world, a returning home with the goods, or the goodies, the core essence—the core qualities that the being incarnated completed creating or developing in the lifetime, therefore having finished the life path and then comes home. Death is a matter of dropping the physical body, which can be looked at as a set of clothes, and moving on to the next phase of your life. One can say it's death in the physical but not the spiritual. One can see it that way, but that is very dualistic. It's simply a transition, and usually quite a happy one, depending on the type of death. After prolonged illness it takes a little longer to regain conscious awareness. A sudden death sometimes is rather disorienting, and as you know, people don't realize they have dropped their body.

"To us, death is simply moving to the next level of growth and creation, and anyone who has chosen to enter into the physical incarnation has also chosen to become a cocreator with the divine. And to have individual free will. Once having chosen that, then you have set yourself up for many spirals of learning that continue infinitely. The key here, perhaps, is that incarnation is considered to be quite painful. And there is a time, then, through your cycles when you realize that incarnation is really about cocreation, then your continued existence as cocreator becomes more and more joyful with each incarnation. One must look at life as a continued spiraling of cocreation with the Divine that becomes more and more pleasurable and is infinite and timeless. When you have gone through a certain amount of duality, you will also have released your dependency on the limitation of so-called linear time. That helps you focus where you need to during the incarnation."

According to Heyoan there is no difference between the spiritual and physical. "What you call 'death' is actually your limited ability at this point in your evolution to understand the true nature of your own being. You would call it a process of losing your body. We would call it simply an expansion of understanding, for the physical is truly as spiritual as what is now called the spiritual and there truly is no separation."

So the connection to God or the Creator, the ultimate connection in life is always there, even though we might feel that it's not. It's just perception. Heyoan is saying, "It is always there, and if one is able to raise one's consciousness to the fourth level, of the field of the astral world, you will immediately make that connection consciously. It never goes away. Your loved ones of course do go through different levels of consciousness, after leaving the body. But that doesn't mean that they are not contactable. Indeed, you are the ones who are difficult to contact."

Heyoan says there are many ways to help after the loss of a loved one. It is here that prayer and ceremony are great gifts to those who have passed on who need such relief. But to us, death is simply an awakening to the greater awareness of being, and from your perspective, shall I say it in dualistic terms, simply dropping the clothes of the physical, or changing the clothes of the physical, or releasing the chain with which you chain yourself, or lock yourself, to the limited view of what the physical actually is."

We each have our own journey in life and the more we understand and honor the cycle of life, which includes death, the more we can fully live and die. After my mother's passing, I had a most blessed gift—one that taught me that there is more to life and death than meets the eye. As my sister and I were exiting the elevator at the L.A. International Airport baggage claim, returning from taking my mother to Santa Monica Hospital in Rosarita Beach, Mexico, I noticed to my left the spiritual presence of my mother and father in living color, very young and from the neck up looking at my sister and myself, with utmost love and compassion. They spoke, although not with their lips, but I could understand them. They said, "Look at what our life was about." They smiled and were in utmost peace. I knew they were referring to raising us three children, and how much love and fulfillment it had given them. In turn, they gifted me with the blessing of knowing they were happy and together. Seeing them was as clear as sitting and talking to my daughter today. They have come to me since in dreams and warned me and inspired me, and each and every time they have greatly affected my life.

Throughout the years, it has been difficult for me to be totally authentic with my brother and sister and other loved ones with my feelings. I have wanted to be in control at least to some degree. To just cry in their arms or to let them cry in mine has been uncomfortable. Today, I am working on sharing what is in my heart and allowing myself to be vulnerable and real. The old pattern in our family, of each withdrawing and feeling separate from one another with our pain, is slowly changing. We are learning to be more honest and true with one another. As we become conscious of this new way of being, we are remembering to be gentle with ourselves and with one another, and to honor each other's process of healing and growing.

Chapter Eight

Reconnecting After Losing a Homeland

"The Wounded Knee memorial ceremony in 1990 was not to forget the past, but to complete ourselves spiritually. And we prayed that there would be no more Wounded Knees throughout the world."   —*Chief Arvol Looking Horse*

Most Americans have never felt the pain and distress of losing their homeland. However, Native Americans understand all too well the hardship and agony of losing their freedom and of being confined to reservations. African Americans as well have faced the harshest of cruelty being stolen from their homeland and subjugated into slavery, and Japanese Americans during World War II experienced tremendous hardship and pain when forcibly removed from their homes into internment camps.

The consciousness of millions of Americans shifted dramatically on September 11, 2001, after the tragic attack on the World Trade

Center and the Pentagon. Suddenly the sacredness of preserving one's homeland became paramount in people's minds and hearts. Many of those who had not previously felt the agony of people across the globe, or for that matter people in their own country, afflicted with violence and oppression, were more sensitive to what millions of people on our planet endure day in and day out.

One of the greatest truths to come out of the recent tragedy is how intensely interdependent we are as a world unit. The world is our homeland, and we must acknowledge our interdependence. A challenge to overcome is to move from an individual consciousness to a collective consciousness and recognize globalization on a spiritual level—that we are all interconnected. Throughout history, people of many cultures and nations have been forced from their homelands for various reasons. This chapter includes different stories from the Native American, Guatemalan, Jewish, and Chilean experiences to see from their point of view what it is like to be exiled and what they have done to heal themselves. It is my hope to convey their pain, their inspiration, and their truths in order that we may learn lessons from them.

Chief Arvol Looking Horse is the nineteenth-generation keeper of the Sacred White Buffalo Calf Pipe, and spiritual leader of the Lakota, Dakota, and Nakota nations. Arvol has carried the awesome responsibility of caring for the sacred bundle of his people since he was twelve years old. In staying connected to the original instructions and spiritual teachings of his people, Arvol shares, "The White Buffalo Calf Woman appeared hundreds of years ago, bringing instructions and sacred ceremonies of how to live in balance with all of life.

She left behind a sacred bundle containing a pipe of peace. She left prophecies about a time in which she would return again. As she came she was singing some songs. Today we still do these ceremonies and sing these same songs."

Although Arvol and his people were given instructions on how to live their lives in a peaceful way, they lived during an era when their spiritual ways were outlawed and mocked.

For Arvol, a major point of transformation in his own healing came about in 1990, during a ceremony called Mending the Sacred Hoop that was for the more than 300 women, children, and elders who were massacred at Wounded Knee in 1890, as well as for the surviving families, who have been hurt in every way possible by this desecration of their relatives and way of life. "Survivors of the relatives participated, as well as people of other nations. Until we went through this ceremony, we were not aware of the level of pain, anger, hatred, and jealousy that we were carrying, all the things that do not belong in the ceremonies. We were instructed that it would take four years of doing the ceremony to fully understand the meaning of the Mending the Sacred Hoop, spirit-releasing ceremony. We rode on horseback like our ancestors, oftentimes at temperatures below forty degrees." Arvol was the spiritual leader of the ride to Wounded Knee, and he says that their ride was not to forget the past but to complete themselves spiritually. They prayed that there would be no more Wounded Knees throughout the world.

The ceremony provided much healing for Arvol and many others. He remembers, "After the ceremony, I felt like I let go of the pain. I felt like I was part of the hoop that was mending. I found peace within myself. Young people rode and learned and grew. From this ceremony, I have been given much guidance and strength to carry on my life's work in helping to create healing and peace for Mother Earth and for all of her relations."

The pain of becoming disenfranchised on his own homeland served as a catalyst for Arvol to begin to educate himself. He grew motivated to learn everything he could about his tribe, his state, and the U.S. government. He remembers, "I began to read more about treaties and the U.S. government. Our elders talked about the reservations that were lived on as concentration camps. Each reservation had a number given to it. The reservation I live on is called Cheyenne River Reservation and it has its own number.

One of the ways to exterminate indigenous people is to take away their food source and livelihood. Arvol's father had provided him with about sixty to seventy cattle and told him that they owned the cattle and the horses. The tribal government, acting on behalf of the U.S. government, came down one day and took everything they had—the cows, horses, and machinery to make their hay. They were left with just a house.

There was also tremendous discrimination and hatred directed toward his people. In 1952 a bill was created called the "Shoot the Indian" bill. Arvol recalls, "The people on the reservations, these concentration camps, were powerless. This had a great effect on me. I was a Lakota man, and I had no place upon Mother Earth, in my home territory of our nation. That was the darkest time in my life. I had nothing. We were left for nothing, and that's why I cried at my grandmother's grave, because I didn't want to go on with my life, because it was not beautiful."

But in keeping connected to the original instructions given by the White Buffalo Calf Woman in carrying out the prayers, ceremonies, and cultural ways, Arvol grew stronger. He learned to feel gratitude and to get along with people of all backgrounds. He began to understand his place in life. His grandfather once said to him, "Today we do our prayers silently, but someday people all over all the world are going to depend on us, because we are the caretakers of the sacred sites, and the caretakers of the sacred bundles. And through this, we are going to help many, many people upon Mother Earth." Arvol was able to keep his connection to the wisdom and teachings passed down to him, and in living his life in accordance to these spiritual principles and way of life, he was able to heal. He says, "Through all the hardships that our people have gone through, we still have our traditional government, our way of life, the ceremonies, and our Sacred Bundle. Our laws are with the Creator. And that's what the Seven Sacred Rites are about that come with the Sacred Bundle."

Today there is still much pain in his people's hearts. The legacy of war and destruction has made its way through the generations. He says, "We're supposed to be a nation that is very strong in spirituality, but we're weakened by what has happened to our relatives before us who have survived the wars. We're in a time of mending the sacred hoop of life. Today we're doing ceremonies more openly to help bring about an understanding of our way of life. That we are not the way a lot of people read about Native Americans in books as savages or people that take scalps. We are a peaceful people. We work toward world peace. What I feel good about is that today there are many ceremonies taking place and people are learning to feel connected to this. It is very beautiful to see. We are once again learning to be healthy and to heal and move through our pain, to let go of the past and to pray for the future."

Similar to Arvol, Nobel Peace Prize Laureate Rigoberta Menchú Tum understands the heartbreak of losing her family, loved ones, and much of her Mayan nation to genocide. She has been forced into exile for a second time, continuing to use her voice to speak out for human rights and for the protection of the natural environment. I had the great honor of being asked by Rigoberta in 1980, shortly after she had been forced to flee her homeland, to be her interpreter and translator at an indigenous people's tribunal in Davis, California. Speaking out on behalf of her lost relatives and the many who have been forced to live under the most brutal of conditions. Her voice helped to change the lives of millions and millions of people within her country, as well as throughout the world.

The pain of growing up feeling connected to one's people and way of life and then suddenly becoming marginalized and disenfranchised, through extreme violence and oppression, creates much heartache and sorrow. Rigoberta remembers, "I was born in a very small town. All the people that lived in Chimel, where I was born, knew each other. When the conflict started in July of '79, some persons were kidnapped; others were assassinated. But the most terrible of all was that my brother Patrocinio was taken. Even he, who was so young when he was kidnapped, was cruelly tortured, and then assassinated.

"Shortly after, my father too was killed. Then some two and a half months later, my mother was kidnapped and was tortured."

Violence and oppression forced Rigoberta to flee her homeland. She felt totally disconnected and uprooted. Not only was she grieving the death of her loved ones and friends, she had to enter into a different world and learn those ways in order to survive. "Perhaps the most difficult moments in my life were the times I was the most active confronting the situation. I can tell you that in my country I never knew what to think about boarding an airplane. I never thought about how to survive in a city, what to do if I missed a train or bus, or how to conduct myself in a city of total strangers. In the village where I was born there were no strangers. Everyone knew who everyone was, how he or she was and their character. But this experience was different."

Rigoberta always had friends who helped her, and when she was exiled to Mexico, she befriended spiritual people, such as nuns and bishops. In this way, Rigoberta began to connect with people across the globe who were concerned with human rights. This gave her life a sense of greater meaning and purpose and assisted her on her healing journey. She wanted to be a humble example so that no one else would have to go through what she endured. Perhaps there is no greater horror and pain than that of the massacre of one's people. As Rigoberta recounts, "I witnessed the massacres of Akxial and the massacres of Xaman. When the massacre of Xaman in Guatemala happened in 1995 I saw the people, the coffins, the people crying, the orphans. At one point I couldn't cry or speak or do anything. There was a moment when all I felt was the solemnity of the place and my anger. I believe I don't have the anger that could overcome all that evil. One seemingly feels powerless."

For Rigoberta, seeking the truth in every situation and sharing the love she has for humanity, the land, and for all of life has nourished and sustained her spirit. What she has grown to believe is, "The conquistadors, the colonizers, did not have any cultural intentions of preserving the lives of the planet's cultures but rather of invading and imposing their agenda. They did a lot of damage in regard to the history they wrote. The history they wrote was not of the people who created, thought, and lived there. But in order to monopolize the resources of the indigenous people, the invaders destroyed the memories of the indigenous people, and the history the colonizers wrote is what is taught everywhere. They created exclusionary systems. But the foundation of humanity, what many people call—and what in our Maya culture we call—'creation,' creation in general is diverse. Creation is multicultural, multiethnic, and multilingual."

People are meant to connect and to feel connected with oneself and with all of the natural creation. Yet how many of us understand the true meaning of being connected?

In today's modern world, it is all too common to feel disconnected from the memory and teachings of our ancestors. Rigoberta understands how to integrate this ancient wisdom and apply it to her life today. "We, the Maya, believe that people are great because we are diverse. We are grand because we are pluralistic. We also are grand because we defend the memory of our elders. We don't want to be like them because we believe that time passes through us according to the time it is our destiny to live. That is, it is not possible for one person to be exactly like another. A person may be the same in some of the characteristics, but not in everything. There is, then, simply a natural rhythm. If people come to love, respect, and admire the culture of another, and admire how another person is, how another culture is, we would truly learn to combat racism."

Perhaps the greatest healing is found in the giving and sharing of oneself. After so much pain and loss, Rigoberta came to realize that "nothing can be greater than the love people have for each other. I have dedicated my life to social causes. I felt I had to finish the work my parents had not finished, their social causes, such as human rights." She is an advocate for people to come together in love and peace.

Rigoberta exemplifies the truth in this in a most extraordinary way. She has experienced the horrific losses of her family and loved ones, and as a result of this violence was forced to leave her homeland. Without a profound sense of feeling rooted and connected to her cultural and spiritual ways, certainly she would not have been able to endure such loss, and advocate so strongly for people to come together in love and peace.

Millions of people on the planet have experienced the pain of being forced to flee their homeland because of the terror of genocide. William Herskovic has endured the pain and horror of the Jewish genocide. As Jews, William, his wife, Esther, and their two young daughters, Kate, four, and Germaine, fourteen months old, were captured by the Nazis while trying to cross the border into unoccupied

France. They were herded into cattle cars at Drancy, with Auschwitz as the destination.

William shares, "We were on the train and we had no food and no drink. It was late August and very hot. It's difficult to understand how it was for my little girl who was fourteen months old and crying and sweating nonstop. She wanted water and she heard somebody urinating into a metal tin and she thought she heard water. She became hysterical. It was terrible. We were on this train for three days and three nights. Locked into this thing. And there was no room to sit or to lie down. We were like cigars standing. Two or three people could sit for about an hour and then they had to let another two or three sit down.

"Then the train stopped in Cosel, east of Germany and not far from Auschwitz. As they opened the wagons, these military police started hitting the people, and yelling for all the men between fifteen and fifty to get out of the wagon. They were screaming that nobody should complain and they ordered us out while they hit people over their heads. People were falling down and everybody was running out, and men were jumping out of the wagon. And when I left, my girls started yelling, 'Daddy, Daddy, don't let me stay here!' I heard them, and I became crazy. Something happened in me. Then a few hours later I asked my friend what happened. I couldn't remember anything. The last thing I heard was my daughters crying."

William was determined to escape the concentration camp to find out if his wife and children were spared the death camps and to tell the world the truth about what was happening to Jews. William planned his escape from the moment he arrived at the camp. He received rubber boots in the camp but hid them to sell them for money to take the train when he escaped. William decided to talk with a head man at the camp who was Czechoslovakian to find out what happened to his wife and daughters. This man told him that the women and children went to the gas chambers right away and that the young people, the strong ones, men and women without children were the only ones with a chance to survive.

This was a turning point for William. He was more determined than ever to escape, even though it was almost unheard of to escape alive from a concentration camp. He says, "I knew I had to escape to find out if there was any chance that my wife and daughters were spared." William eventually escaped and ended up in Belgium. He remembers going to a rabbi and telling the rabbi what was going on only to have the rabbi say, " 'It's not as bad as you think. I have a brother and I received two postcards from him from a camp.' I said, 'He, like others, is forced to write and say that everything is OK and that is not the truth.' "

An integral part of William's healing from such tragic loss was to be able to tell his story. What gave his life meaning was to help others avoid the pain and torment he went through.

The legacy of speaking one's truth and coming together with others to share a message of peace and unity was carried through one of William's grandsons. Together with other grandchildren of grandparents who had experienced different forms of genocide, Native American, African American, Japanese American, Mexican American, and Jewish American children are telling the stories of their grandparents in a film that is being distributed to over 44,000 schools.

When we are true to ourselves and do what we are moved to do, regardless of the circumstances, our efforts reach out to more people than we may ever dream possible. Such was the case with William, and as an elder he continues to move and inspire people to tell their truth and to come together with each other's pain and injustices, and to heal by listening to one another and coming together as one. Through the extreme violence William has been witness to, he has learned that walls built to separate people based on race, economics, or any other reason are unhealthy for humankind. His heart was broken open to the possibility of celebrating diversity and discovering our oneness. William has learned the lessons of perseverance, speaking his truth, learning to move on without forgetting his loved ones, and standing up for what he believes in.

In much the same way as William, Isabel Allende endured the onslaught of bloodshed and terror that occurred during the 1973 military coup in Chile. In a short time, her life changed forever when her family was targeted in the political battle and exiled to Venezuela. She remembers being very angry and feeling total loss. She says, "I was mourning for my country, and mourning for my family and everything that I had lost. It was a very bad time, a very confusing time in my life. And I had the feeling that I was swirling, like a crazy dervish, whirling and nothing had any meaning, I couldn't succeed in anything. Everything was a failure. I couldn't find a job. I did all sorts of odd jobs to make a living, but there was nothing that was creative, or nothing that was meaningful to me."

Oftentimes we can only see in hindsight that our losses may have indeed been preparing us for our most meaningful life's work. For Isabel, she says, "I lost my extended family, my home, my job, my friends, and my country. From that sense of loss came my writing. I didn't know then that I was beginning to create a universe of my own, that is my country. There is that fictional world, in which my characters live, and in which I dwell ten hours a day. And book after book, word by word, I have enlarged this creation of this universe, this fictional universe in which I feel that I belong. And so, it has become more complex, with more characters, and more people—it's like a village, inhabited by so many different people! And that is where my roots are."

In her writing, Isabel has gained much insight and learned many lessons about who she is and what is important to her. "I wrote *The House of the Spirits* to recover a world that I had lost and in writing the book what I healed was the sense of exile, the paralyzing homesickness of the exiles. I realized in a way that I had created a country that was this book and I could carry it with me. A country where I lived, it was a country of my own creation, my imagination, but it was so real to me that it was as real as Chile had been before. It took years for me to realize and to understand that each book was part of a healing process, each book was like a stage in my life that corresponded to something that had happened that usually was painful. The book was a way of feeling my pain, and of transforming the pain into something different."

In time, Isabel was able to come to terms with her own anger and with all of her losses. From this she was able to learn many important lessons. She says, "It's not that the anger was gone because it's never gone, but I could understand it better. And I also learned a very important lesson. I learned that the people who suffered the most, the people who had been tortured, who had lost children to torture, whose members of their families had disappeared, people who had seen the mutilated bodies of their relatives by torture were less angry than I was. They never spoke of revenge, they never said I want to torture the torturer. I want to rape the rapist, I want to kill the killer. They wanted to understand, they wanted to bury their dead. They were not looking for revenge, because in a way revenge is not healing. They were doing what needed to be done, and that was to understand where the horror came from."

Being forced to move into another country can be extremely disorienting. It can be difficult to establish a feeling of connectedness or rootedness when one has become disconnected and uprooted from their land of origin. "When I moved to the United States I felt that I had moved onto a different planet, with a new language, new people, and a different set of codes, rules, and ethics. It was very difficult, but from that sense of starting anew, I gained a new strength that has been very important to me in my life. Now I know I could live anywhere. I could live in a tent in the desert and I would be OK."

Isabel has learned firsthand what it means to live among extreme violence and oppression. From that experience she cherishes even more being able to live in peace. Feeling connected to the rest of humanity and all living things, she has come to believe in the idea of creating a world without war. "We could find a way of having peace in the world, if we could by this accumulated notion of pain, get together and say we know what war is and we know what war does. We have to avoid it. We've learned this but we don't apply this understanding as a collective. Perhaps that is why we continue to walk in circles and we keep stumbling on the same stones."

Pain is a great teacher, when we are willing to learn the lessons it can teach us. Isabel believes that pain can put us in touch with something about ourselves that we're unaware of. She believes that because of what she has gone through she knows her true limitations and her true strengths. In healing and transforming her pain, Isabel has become aware of the truth that we are both interconnected and interdependent. She elaborates, "I'm aware all of the time that there is something that is me that is not visible that is not this person you see on the inside or the outside. It's like a particle of the common spirit that exists for everything and everybody and I say everything because I am an atomist. I really think that trees and stones and rivers and everything have a spirit too, and are part of the same spirit. I believe that this particle of spirit that I carry is indestructible and my job in this world is to accumulate experience and knowledge for that particle of spirit to be enriched when it reunites with a common spirit. It goes back to a sort of ocean of consciousness and my job is to contribute to that ocean by using my lifetime and my body and my senses and my imagination and my work and whatever, to contribute to that. But this is something that I have learned at fifty-five. As a young person I really believed that I was an individual, and that being an individual was important; I don't think that anymore."

Isabel inspires us in her ability to reconnect through planting her roots in her memory and in her books. Those are her connections. This has given her the ability to give back to this country. She says, "I try to serve as much as possible and to give back, because I receive a lot. I created a foundation after my daughter died. I give back to refugees and I give back to women and children. Not only in the United States, but I give back in Central America, in Chile, and in India. This is my greatest joy right now."

Still today, Lenny Foster is witnessing the devastation and breakdown of his people caused by their forced removal from their homelands and health crises they endure due to uranium and coal strip mining of their land. Lenny is a spokesperson for the Dineh (Navajo) at the United Nations as well as other global gatherings, and is a spiritual advisor for Native American inmates in the prison system.

Forced relocation causes much suffering for anyone, and it is even more painful when a people's entire way of life, culture, and religion are based on living in communion with the spirit of their land. Lenny laments, "There are four sacred mountains that border our indigenous territories, our homelands, where we believe we originated from. On the Eastern boundary is Mt. Blanca. On the southern boundary is Mt. Taylor. The Western boundary is the San Francisco Peaks, and the northern boundary is called Mt. Hesparua. We believe that we originated from four sacred mountains that surround our homelands and these lands are very sacred to our people. We live in a traditional way with the land, raising our livestock and growing plants for our survival, such as corn, potatoes, squash, melons, and apples.

"That is the way that many of our people lived. When our ancestors were forcibly removed from their land, they had to endure a 'long walk,' relocating from Fort Defiance to Fort Sumner. This relocation 'walk' lasted five years and it was one of the most debilitating psychological and emotional experiences our people ever faced. In retelling this historical event, our elders taught us the need to remember what took place in those years. People were imprisoned without trial for years. Eventually, a treaty was signed with the U.S. government in 1868, which allowed us to return to our homelands in what is now part of New Mexico, Arizona, and Utah.

"Our homeland is more than merely a place where we are born. It encompasses all aspects of life woven into the spiritual, emotional, mental, physical, cultural, and economic life of our people. When people are forced off their homeland, they become disconnected and fragmented. A second forced relocation policy affecting the Dineh people began in the 1960s."

Lenny explains further, "Once more the U.S. government is in the process of forcibly moving our people off their lands in the Big Mountain, Nebatoe, and Hard Rock areas. The Dineh people are resisting this forced relocation, but they are being placed on a track of land in Flagstaff and other nearby border towns, and suffering severely. I think it brings back the meaning of the resistance our ancestors went through when they were forcibly relocated on that 'long walk.' This is devastating because we are connected to our spiritual origin through our legends and stories, and through the land where our ancestors are buried. Consequently we consider forced displacement of our community to be cultural genocide."

Lenny explains, "We have very strong ties to the land and we consider it to be sacred. We feel that we are one with the plants and animals that live on the land. The genocide that is taking place is due to exposure to hazardous mining waste, state initiated conflicts, and disempowerment. Our people were never told about the hazardous effects uranium mining would have on us. No one told us about the radioactive tailings from the waste that was left behind and never cleaned up from the radioactive pollution. So people used the radioactive tailings to build their homes and children played on what appeared to be sand dunes. The radioactive tailings also got into the water supply and now the people and livestock have to drink this water. The water table is being depleted as well as the air being polluted and the people and animals in this region are getting sick. And some of the plants no longer grow. These poisons affect not only people who live in the immediate area, but also people and living things who live where the winds and rivers carry these known carcinogens in the natural cycle of life. Many of our people have died from cancer or are suffering the effects of cancer. I feel that the U.S. government has denied responsibility and the consequences of what is happening to our people and our land. And any kind of restitution is delayed or opposed."

Lenny, along with his people, has suffered and endured the harshest circumstances caused by losing their homeland. In his anguish he went to his elders for guidance. He began a spiritual journey following the Sun Dance way as well as attending the Native American church and began to learn how to release and heal his sorrow. Against all odds, he learned to convert an overwhelming sense of powerlessness and discover his calling as a spokesperson for his people. He has also found a mission in working with the Dineh and other indigenous inmates who have not found the means to transform their pain. During Lenny's healing, he has truly learned the meaning of reconnecting after the loss of one's homeland.

Chief Arvol Looking Horse, Rigoberta Menchú Tum, William Herskovic, Isabel Allende, and Lenny Foster have each had their unique experiences with loss of homeland, but all have learned from their respective journeys. They have each gained a greater appreciation of who they are and how to remain true to themselves. The first step in stopping oppression and the taking over of lands that don't belong to us is to realize that we are a global world. We have the power to make responsible choices and to carry forth with our actions what is healthy for all of life.

Chapter Nine

*"All humanity is one undivided and indivisible family, and
each one of us is responsible for the misdeeds of all the others."*
—Mahatma Gandhi

As a young person, I often felt that I did not belong. It was not
until I was twenty-seven and sitting in a Native American sweat
lodge, in a circle facing the glistening rocks, burning cedar, sage, and
sweetgrass, that I truly felt at home. I was one with the elements,
huddled close to others in total darkness, listening to the prayers,
song, drum, and the voice coming from my heart. For the first time I
felt as if I were with other people who shared my concerns, visions,
and pain. Together we experienced a deep reverence and love for
Mother Earth and for all of natural creation. I felt what it meant to
be part of a community. Honoring and blessing these sacred gifts in

ourselves and one another benefits the whole community. And when healthy communities make up the world, we are re-creating the world.

After this ceremony, I began to realize that the healthier we are as individuals and families, the healthier our communities are. I recognized that so many communities break down because people place greater value on acquiring material goods to give them happiness, rather than coming together and sharing one another's stories, perceptions, and experiences in life to find fulfillment. A kind of rugged individualism develops from this overly materialistic way of life, leaving people feeling separated and isolated from one another.

The loss of community is an inevitable result of having to work longer and harder in order to purchase more things. Often people are too tired and stressed to get together, and what time they do spend is usually with immediate family or friends. Most people choose to watch their TV, go on their computer, watch a DVD or video, or entertain themselves alone or with a few persons they are close with. Little time is spent in nature.

In modern culture, generations are separated where elders and children have little interaction in the community. Activities are stratified according to age, providing little interaction and much confusion and misunderstanding between the generations.

Our community is a mirror of who we are individually and as families. So many of us have felt disconnected from ourselves and our family that we have yet to learn what it means to give to and to receive.

In transforming our pain, we can move from our numbness, rage, and anger back to the original hurt we have been carrying, and in recognizing and feeling what our pain is, connect with our higher selves and make choices that are conscious and loving. Communities re-created from this consciousness will certainly bring about more healing and joy.

We have models of communities where kindness and generosity are valued more than a person's accumulated wealth. People nurture and care for one another, creating loving and safe neighborhoods. It is no great mystery to know how to live in harmony with ourselves and one another when that is our purpose.

I have been very moved by people who live close to the land and who remember their spiritual traditions. They are humbled and strengthened living in harmony with nature. My experiences walking across the United States on the Longest Walk, living on the Native American reservations, in Latin America, and traveling to South Africa have reminded me that there are still communities in the world where people feel connected, nurtured, and loved.

It is up to us to decide whether we wish to once again learn what that means. We all know someone from an older generation or another culture who remembers what it is like to feel connected to their community. We can learn from their experiences and shape communities that serve our needs of today, while embracing our true potential as human beings capable of leaving a healthy and joyful legacy for the future generations to come.

I have been greatly inspired by the life stories, perceptions, and experiences of many people in learning to re-create community. They have reminded me of the resiliency of the human spirit, and each has chosen to give back to the community their insights and under-standing of the gift of pain.

While I was in South Africa, a dear friend, Afrika Msimang, shared with me an IsiZulu description of community. This speaks to the global heart of humanity.

"Ubuntu is an IsiZulu term which means *humanness.* This con-cept can be described as a political foundation of all African societies. It is a unifying vision enshrined in an IsiZulu proverb 'umuntu agu-muntu ngabanye,' meaning one is a person through others." One of her very dear elders, Ntate Koka, an African sage, sums up a com-munity as follows: "The philosophy of humanness, imbued with in-finite love, makes us as individuals within the community—to feel, see, and recognize our 'being,' our very existence, efforts, success, and failures, interests, ambitions, and aspirations, in other members of the community. We, as individuals, and the community become fused into each one of us."

Afrika Msimang was born and raised in Soweto, South Africa, and at the age of seven witnessed the massacre of hundreds of children in her community by the apartheid regime. She has worked as a media liaison officer in the post-apartheid South African National Parlia-ment, a journalist on *The Argus* newspaper, a media officer on Robben Island, and a co-director of the Parliament of the World's Religions, hosted in South Africa. Additionally, she is studying to qualify as a Montessori teacher.

Afrika grew up in a township, a community created by the

apartheid regime to prevent Africans from becoming self-sufficient. She believes that, "the African way of life has a social ethic, a unifying vision enshrined in the IsiZulu maxim, 'one is a person through others.' As a child I understood this enlightened way of life during funerals and weddings. These occasions cemented relationships and friendships. During such times people reached out of themselves and found fulfillment and nurturing. In giving, they received. In our culture there were no orphans, because of the nature of the extended family. However, subtle individualistic tendencies have been slowly eroding our culture in the past few decades."

A community can be made stronger when it is faced with adversity. Afrika shares, "I grew up in a very rooted community and a relatively stable home. Our community was united against the common evils of colonization—subjugation, degradation, and poverty. Laws were promulgated to separate us into tribal groups, but we resisted such micro-identification."

Perhaps the greatest pain a parent can face is having to leave their own children. In Soweto, Afrika says, "Most of our parents worked as domestic workers in a divided South Africa. They fed and clothed European children and would return home to their children on weekends or once a month. Their children were forced to look after themselves at a tender age. At the age of eight, my sister was able to prepare dinner for the family. Most children's fathers worked as laborers in the mines. That meant seeing their fathers once a year during Christmas."

Within the moral fabric of Afrika's family, her mother taught the children to regard all elders in the area as parents, to be treated with respect. "When I was nine years old, our elderly neighbor was involved in a car accident. She underwent surgery and was returned home too soon. We could not trace her daughters and we had to look after her. I was obliged to check on her every morning before school and after school and before bedtime. That included cleaning her house and attending to her. My sister included her in all the meal preparations. The arrangement went on for a very long time before one of her daughters finally visited her."

Regardless of outside influences, our parents have the greatest impact on our belief system and how we behave towards others. For Afrika, her mother instilled values in her that have fostered a great sense of community. "My mother's inclusive and compassionate way of life made me believe in the essence of communalism. Her many unspoken lessons taught me that sharing is an act of grace. At the age of twelve I started visiting the orphanage in Orlando, some nine kilometres from my house. I had no ambition to dramatically change the quality of anyone's life, nor the vocabulary to express my pleasure to spend time with parentless children. When I first arrived there, the caretakers seemed surprised but were happy to have me around. I spent many of my Saturday afternoons playing with infants and feeding toddlers."

Afrika grew to understand that she was a child of the struggle. "We have an African history that predates the emergence of Europe. As a youth growing up in an apartheid South Africa, I was denied the pleasure of understanding where I came from and there were many obstacles to prevent the community from moving forward. As the saying goes, 'if you do not know where you come from, you shall never know where you are going to.' I was not going to be stopped from fighting for our emancipation as well as embarking on the journey of excavating my authentic self.

"We, the youth, had adopted a policy of liberation before education. It made schooling difficult, but it was an essential vehicle towards attaining our freedom. We honored the call of the struggle as well as continued with apartheid education. We have emotional, physical, and intellectual scars to show the road we have traveled.

"Ironically, it was the struggle against colonization that encouraged us to work together as a team, and yet many centuries of struggling against lack of social justice and human rights have slowly eroded our moral fiber as a community. High levels of cultural imperialism have robbed us of our humanity. Sadly, we are undermining our hard-earned liberation with the loss of the community and moral values."

Afrika emphasizes that, "There is a missing link between a rooted African culture, spirituality, and education in our country. The cultural and moral collapse was encouraged and driven by the colonial powers. Today, people in the Western world are grappling with new paradigms to understand their role in society, while most Africans continue to be fascinated by the very culture most spiritually centered Westerners are trying to discard—the culture of rugged individualism completely devoid of ubuntu."

Leaders in a community can have a great influence on its people. This was the case for Afrika and so many millions of South Africans. "Our leaders have shown us that forgiveness frees us. I had to learn to forgive the settlers who invaded my country and continent and robbed us of our humanity. I had to learn to forgive myself for having moments of African pessimism, the 'Nothing Can Be Done Syndrome,' and for my impatience with the world. It has been a long journey and a graceful experience. This act of forgiveness has helped me to heal at a core level. I have come to realize that it is not all lost in the African culture, we can rebuild our community. In one of his most eloquent speeches, our President, Thabo Mbeki, has urged us 'To sketch a landscape in which to act out our collective dream and to fabricate a plan to deliver us from the consequences of our human weakness.' "

The actions of Tata Nelson Mandela have inspired Afrika to learn to forgive. "Tata Nelson Mandela demonstrates the courage it takes for a victim to forgive his or her perpetrators. After twenty-seven years of incarceration, he walked out of prison with a smile and a clenched fist, vigorously waving to the multitude of people. Tata Mandela went to the extent of visiting the widow of the architect of apartheid for tea at her house in Oranje, a suburb in the Western Cape Province, that is desperately trying to perpetuate segregation. He has called on South Africans to heal the divisions of the past and to establish a new society which observes fundamental human rights."

Afrika reminds us that through adversity we are given the opportunity to excavate our true self and honor what our soul longs for. When we remember the truth of who we are and where we come from, we are strengthened and given the ability to co-create with others a profound sense of community.

When he was honorary mayor of Malibu, California, Martin Sheen was not afraid to stand up for what he believes in. He spoke about making the community a "protective zone for all of life—humans and wild." That was his last act as honorary mayor. Martin has experienced the pain of having conflicting values with many of his neighbors over what is socially conscious, ecologically sound, and morally right. When we speak our truth, we may pay a price, but we carry an even greater burden when we don't share what is in our hearts.

In Martin's efforts to bring about change, he wanted his neighbors to take an honest look at themselves and change some of the local laws. He says, "I tried to show the community itself by holding up a mirror and displaying its true nature and I got scorned. I didn't realize they'd take me seriously. We got some real gutter mail. That incident brought out the worst in people. There was one young couple who wouldn't sign their name but said to me in a vulgar letter how I had devalued their property by my activism and how they had worked all their lives to move here but that I was flushing that down the toilet. I was talking about the value of other human beings, and the environment! But that was not their area of concern. So it was a joke and the joke was on me. And I took a beating."

At times when we are experiencing opposition, it may appear as if everything is going wrong and that our actions have no real significance. It is important to consider that although we may not be able to see the gift of the pain we are feeling, in time when all is revealed, we will understand that there was a meaning and purpose for it all. Martin discovered this. "After that whole incident, I left standing. I had no hard feelings. I'm very honest about the community, they know me, and they know from whence I come. They're very wary of me and very tolerant of me in a lot of cases. A few neighbors agree with me and there are some really good and decent people here who supported me. And as a result, we were able to get liberal and very compassionate feedback which was heretofore unrealized. I was grateful to be the instrument even though I got flushed away in the interim. It was a fascinating time. I wouldn't want to go through it again, but I wouldn't change the experience for the world."

Martin was able to find people from his community of Malibu, California, with similar values, and together they have stood up for issues that deeply concern them. "We began to protest over nuclear testing. They've been testing close to here since the start of the Cold War. They were doing aboveground testing up until the late 1950s. Then they realized that wasn't such a hot idea, because it was destroying the environment. So they decided to start underground testing, and they did that right up until a few years ago. We used to go to the testing site and protest that this is not a good idea for the environment or for the spiritual environment of ourselves as a community. So whenever we knew a test was going to occur, we gathered at the test site and we demonstrated for what we believed in. A great solidarity and sense of community grew from us coming together and standing up for what we believe in."

Martin was looking to re-create his community as a more concerned and active influence for the well-being of everyone. Much like Martin, Isabel Allende learned the significance of re-creating her community in new ways. She shares, "Writing is where my roots are now, and that is where my greatest connections are. After twenty years of writing, I realized that every single book has reached thousands or millions of people. And I am connected to those people. It's like a message in a bottle that I put into the sea. And I never know who will pick it up. There is this network of invisible connections that connects me to people all over the world of all ages and diverse languages."

Isabel is from a culture where extended family and community are extremely important. "In Eastern society or in any primitive society, people are connected to the fact that life works in cycles. That everything is connected. That there's no such a thing as 'disposable.' Everything is recycled in nature, and in the spirit world as well. Everything you do has consequences, there's an effect for everything, for every intention. For every word. In Western society, there is this idea that we can control everything. That there is no destiny, no karma, that there are self-made people is an absurd idea, because we are the result of so many influences. Nobody is self-made. Nobody is alone. Community is what is important, being part of a chain is what is important in life."

Isabel understands the idea of giving and receiving as distinguished from taking. She shares, "Many people expect the community to provide them with certain things. And they never ask themselves, What am I going to give back to the community? They don't question their role in the community. And I think that giving is very important. My feeling of belonging to the community is not from what I get from it. It's about what I can give to it."

Recognizing how pain can act as a catalyst for the transformation of consciousness frees us. Isabel elaborates, "I think that pain puts you in touch with something about yourself that was not recognized before. Through that experience you know better who you are. I know my limitations today and I know my strengths. I know what I can do and what I can't do. I know what I want to do and what I'm not interested in doing, and I don't waste time anymore because I know better the person I am. I have a practical consciousness of the person I am and I have a spiritual consciousness of the spiritual resources I have."

Giving back to others in a nurturing and supportive manner helps to heal our pain. Isabel witnessed this with her mother. "My mother went through a very dark and long depression. She dressed in black and looked old and sick all the time. She went to therapy and was on medication. Nothing helped her. My mother was a rather self-centered person when she went back to live in the democratic Chile of today. An old school friend convinced her to work in some literary workshops with women in the poorest neighborhoods of Santiago who were almost illiterate. Her job was to inspire them to tell their stories.

"She met with these women once a week and in six months my mother was another human being. She forgot about her depression. The stories of those fifteen women haunted her, were with her, and she became part of their story. She got so involved that her depression left. In the process she learned to give her pain boundaries, and she gained greater perspective. For these women this was the first time since the dictatorship and the brutality that someone had listened to their stories."

Isabel had an awakening about the transformative power of connecting with others and sharing our stories. She shares, "The most extraordinary moment was when I returned to Chile for the first time since the coup and my mother said, 'I want you to meet the people from my workshop.' And I went to this poor neighborhood and sat with these women and they were telling me about their lives. They all said, 'No one ever asked our story, no one ever wanted to know what had happened. It was such a long time that I had not talked to anybody that I started to believe that it wasn't true, that it never happened.' As they started to give their accounts in the workshop, sharing it with the other women, it all became real again."

Isabel understands that community is about sharing one another's stories and learning to listen, support, and nurture each other. She has learned that when we share our wisdom, knowledge, and love we help each other. She also reminds us that spending quiet time alone, in prayer and meditation, is extremely important. Sharing the insights and lessons learned strengthens us all.

Joan Borysenko has also felt the loss of community and the need to recreate a new circle she feels connected to. As a child Joan found a sense of roots in Zionist camps. She shares, "I completely loved the ritual. I loved the song and dance. And I was born in 1945, so the state of Israel and I are about the same age. As a child of ten, Israel was a very young country, and we were kind of infused with a sense that there was a homeland for our people who had been scattered across the face of the earth in such an enormous Diaspora.

"Unfortunately I couldn't find in the temple at home the kind of spiritual connection that I'd had as a child at camp. That was probably the greatest disconnection of my life. This sense that somewhere within Judaism there was ritual, there was a place where women belonged, and there was a deep sense of spirituality. Knowing that this was true and not being able to find it outside of the camp in organized Judaism was a terrible blow for me. I then left anything having to do with Judaism."

As Joan grew older she searched for a spiritual community. "I spent seven very wonderful years in a spiritual community, which was actually founded by a Sufi healer who became a mystical Christian. My seven years with that group was my deepest sense of homecoming in early adulthood."

But after Joan's family moved, she was again looking to reconnect with another spiritual community. She found community within a Hindu group, but eventually turned away from her guru, or spiritual leader. "That completely shook the foundation of my universe. The pain was so extraordinarily deep, because I thought, does this invalidate all the spiritual teachings? This made me question the very foundations of my faith.

"I asked myself, what is this, sign up for a cult? Do I have absolutely no discernment? Why did I put myself in that situation? And what is it in me that wants to give my power over to a guru? I got stuck on that point, for a very, very, VERY long time."

During most of her time in this community, Joan shared "at a deep level, psychologically, spiritually, we were having fun together, doing things, and going to India together. And the loss of that group of people, and the divisiveness that occurred in the group following the fall of the guru, was terrible. So that was, of my adult life, the greatest sense of rootlessness and pain."

For Joan, as for many people, not having a spiritual community causes much pain. She shares, "We have our Native American community, but we don't see them all that frequently. And there's the Jewish renewal community in Boulder, but because of my travel schedule, I'm very peripheral to that. I have a somewhat large loose community of people, who I see all over the country a couple times a year, but here in my hometown I don't have a firm root to tap into."

Joan understands the importance of having a personal sense of rootedness. "I feel like I'm the matriarch of my family. I feel a tremendous sense of responsibility for nourishing my family. I'm always trying to figure out what the family rituals are and how I will get people together, because they're scattered across the country. I wonder what are the modern day rituals that will supplant those older rituals of Sunday dinners, when everybody grew up and lived in the same place?

"Another sense of rootedness I have is with the spiritual community that I see a couple of times a year at speaking engagements and conferences. Still another sense of community I have is the intellectual community, and that probably comes from my background as an academic. There can be a strong root in your academic field in terms of the people who went before you, the researcher tradition that you were trying to carry on, your ability to mentor the people who came after you, and in that sense I feel myself as part of a lineage. And that gives me a sense of roots."

Jack Canfield also embarked on a spiritual path that led him to recognize the importance of community. Sometimes in life we are so numbed that we don't know that we are missing out on anything. Jack moved so often that he never felt he was part of a community. "The way I dealt with the pain was to study all the time. And as long as I was studying I was distracted. I read voraciously, went to graduate school, and just kept real busy. I didn't know what I was missing on feeling connected to like-minded people, until I met this guy who invited me to a lecture series on campus. I ended up going, and I liked the tone of the people there and I liked who they were. They felt alive and interesting."

Today, Jack says, "A sense of community is something I'm working on creating right now. In fact, we're starting to create a couples group here in Santa Barbara, conscious couples, getting together on some kind of regular basis. I also feel connected to the spiritual community, my meditation center, and I feel connected to the larger community of Santa Barbara, because it's really a pretty conscious place. There are a lot of people here who really care about the ecology, about not overpopulating the area, about having the community be multicultural and tolerant. And it's a kind of community where a lot of wonderful things are happening. I get invited to functions, and I'm a member of committees, and there are charities that I'm involved with, so I feel connected. That is an important part of community.

"I think people are looking to feel more connected to community. Perhaps one of the reasons for the success of our *Chicken Soup* books has been that they speak to community, because they are self-identifying, like cancer survivors, gardeners, sports fans, and battered mothers. People have common interests and concerns. And so there's a natural built-in connectedness because of mutual concerns and the mutual need to understand things. We've become a focal point, if you will, for people to come together that care about the things that our books talk about, which are living your dreams, love, more emotional openness, vulnerability, family, values, and all of those kinds of things."

Jack is an inspiration in demonstrating how we each can live our dreams and keep our connection to one another in doing so. He also illustrates how when we live our dreams we stay aligned with the truth of who we are and what we are here to do. With that comes abundance and well-being.

Gerry Jampolsky began his spiritual practice because he was feeling isolated and alone and in much pain and distress. Through Gerry's own healing he has been able to share with others his understanding, insights, and wisdom.

Gerry founded The Center for Attitudinal Healing to serve as a sort of community for those struggling with illness. "I was making rounds at U.C. Medical Center, and a seven-year-old child who was dying of cancer asked the oncologist, 'What's it like to die?' And the doctor changed the subject. That got me to thinking about where kids go for information about death and dying. They oftentimes ask the cleaning lady who's mopping up the floor, just to have an honest discussion with someone.

"When I started The Center for Attitudinal Healing, I didn't realize I was also trying to heal myself, and I didn't realize that I was creating a community, with an extended family. Today the Center is located in Sausalito, California, and there are about 150 additional centers or groups in approximately thirty countries throughout the world. With this large community we have an international meeting with 300 to 500 people who attend every other year. People with catastrophic illnesses have been brought together, and children who are suffering loss. But half of the work is helping people who just want to incorporate attitudinal healing in their own lives. We have a community I feel very connected to. We all have the common goal of having peace of mind. So it's a community that's always there to help other people, and to reach out to each other and feel our inner connection. In a sense what we're doing is healing the illusion that we are separate."

How extraordinary that Gerry and his wife Diane Cirincione have devoted so much of their lives to assisting others in learning how to have peace of mind. By healing our attitudes, we are able to re-create healthy communities.

Larry Dossey has discovered that taking time for inner reflection, prayer, and meditation, as well as outward socializing and connecting with others, helps to create balance and harmony. With these attributes we are able to contribute more to recreating our communities.

As we grow, we may change communities. Oftentimes the transition from one community to another is painful and challenging. Larry says, "I've never felt as if I didn't have a community. I've always had a community to support me. What happens however is that the community shifts. There are all sorts of communities. And I've always been supported by some sort of community at each phase of my life. It's painful transitioning from one sort of community to another. There's that little in-between phase where you feel adrift, but if you follow your truth, then other communities that are even more supportive open up and embrace you. That's what I have found. For example, when I was in medical practice, and felt myself being weaned away from a completely physically oriented view on life to one that had a place for consciousness and spirituality, I developed a rich network of scholars around the world who were actually doing the same thing. We wrote, we visited at seminars, we talked on the phone, and we helped each other get through painful transitions. And we supported each other with rejection from the former community that we'd been part of. And so this non-local distant network, in recent years, has been much more important to me than any local community where people gather physically."

People need different kinds of communities. The important thing is to be conscious of our own personal needs for community and to honor and embrace whatever that is. Larry says, "My community now is scattered all over the earth. It's much more sustaining than any other kind of local community ever was. This is different for everybody, though. There's some people who need to get together at sundown and talk with neighbors who are next door. They want a physically localized community. I've never needed that very much, but we have to understand that people's temperaments and personalities are really different, and this makes tremendous differences in the kind of communities we need.

"I'm a hopeless introvert, and I could thrive on distant, non-local, distributed communities. Whereas, I know extroverts who absolutely crave human contact. I can get it in other ways and feel nourished."

In re-creating communities, seeking balance between inward reflection and outward expression is important. Larry shares, "I think that every individual has a need, both for physical connectedness with other people and also for solitude. And I think it's possible to overdo community. Because a lot of people use community as an excuse not to do their personal work. For example, I believe we have in us both the need to unite and to disconnect. And there are moments when we have to go inside and be alone and confront, whatever it is that we are working on. So, one can wean out of doing that sort of work by saying, well I just need to be with people all the time, I need community, community, community. It can be overdone. We have to honor both sides of who we are."

Larry is not afraid to explore who he is and what best serves his needs. In being honest with himself he has successfully re-created a community of people across the globe who he feels extremely connected to and supported by. He inspires us to follow our truth and know that, when we do, the right people will come into our lives.

In a similar way to Larry, Rabbi Zalman Schachter-Shalomi has embraced people from throughout the world, of diverse cultures and ethnicities. His community is made up of his spiritual community at home, as well as those who are like-minded around the world.

"People who belong to a religious community, when they come into a town, will immediately check out their church, or their synagogue, or place of prayer, to find a place where they can find people with whom they can relate. About this I feel very blessed. All the places where I came to, sooner or later there were groups of compatible people with whom I could have an exchange, and collaboration, an extended family."

Social mobility makes it more challenging to feel as if we are part of a community. Rabbi Zalman shares, "I have children all over the place. Some in Israel. Some in Canada. Some in the United States. So, when you see the kind of spread that we have, you can either rely on the blood bonds that you have with relatives, or you have to create communities of people with whom you have the kind of quasi-family relationship.

"So, for instance, when I was sick in the hospital and Eve was looking after me in so many ways, there was a point where she needed some respite. And there were members of the community who provided that. For a couple of weeks people came in and cooked to lend us support. And they are doing the same thing for other people. There is a sense that if there is a bereavement, people in the community pull together to make it easier on the family."

Different traditions have their own ways of helping one another during the death of a loved one. Rabbi Zalman shares, "We have a custom in Jewish community, that when someone dies, you don't let the undertaker prepare the body. It's members of the community that wash the body, dress it in the shroud, and do the last honors. And so it goes from the cradle to the grave, that community comes together. And when you come and you participate in the community, you build that kind of lateral connection, which replaces the bonds that you lost from family."

Rabbi Zalman has a strong sense of what it means to be a global community. He explains, "Sometimes you go and watch a powwow and you're there like a spectator. And sometimes you go and you're not there like a spectator. You hold this field, you send in energy, you participate, you let yourself be taken where it's taking you. And somehow the fact that you're not of the same tribe doesn't matter.

"Once I attended a Native American Sun Dance. There was an elder sitting on the side, telling the men of the Sun Dance the next thing they should do. At one point, he nods over in my direction, and tells the younger man that he should invite me to carry the pipe to a circle, because he had a sense that I wasn't there just gawking. Now, that kind of invitation makes a great deal of difference, y'know?

Rabbi Zalman demystifies the illusion of separation between people of diverse spiritual practices. He shares, "When I was in Calgary, I was up on the roof saying my prayers, and a Mud Indian, Native Canadian, came up there, saying his prayers. We both greeted the dawn over the prairie with prayer, and then shared with one another our sacred implements."

It is so heartwarming when our spiritual leaders of today embody the understanding of our connectedness and oneness as human beings. Rabbi Zalman inspires people wherever he goes, because he understands what it means to have a global heart.

Dr. Deepak Chopra also understands that re-creating community is about accepting people for their unique gifts and diversity. Deepak is a best-selling author of many books, founder of the Chopra Center for Well Being, and a world-famous speaker. The Chopra Center for Well Being brings together people from all walks of life from across the globe. He has carried a vision of how to re-create community that is committed to the health and wellness of the people who come to the Center.

Our upbringing can shape how we view the world. For Deepak, his family structure and upbringing helped to give him the rootedness and understanding of what this Center was to be. He shares, "I come from a strong family structure and support family in the form of cousins, uncles, aunts, and then extended family. I always look at my patients as my extended family. I have never felt that there was a lack of community. It just kept growing larger and larger."

In re-creating community, it is important to take into consideration the needs and wishes of the members. The Center for Well Being attracts many kinds of people. In Deepak's words, "Some people come to the Chopra Center for Well Being because they're in pain and suffering. A lot of people come because they're actually doing extremely well, and they're seeking to extend their intuition and creativity and vision and their connection with the sacred. I think in fact the majority of people who come here are not in pain; they are actually in transformation to higher and expanded states of consciousness.

"We focus on four areas in particular: health, spirituality, relationships, and success. And the community has grown. Now we have a discussion board on our Internet site which is called 'My Potential,' and again we have discussion boards on all these four areas. We have a prayer circle with over 12,000 participants. And it's growing by a few hundred every day. So the community keeps expanding, and it's a worldwide community. There is much thought about why we are not more conscious as a community of human beings on the planet. The fact is today we have the most evolved society that has ever existed. And it hasn't evolved because we are praying more or meditating more. The only reason it's evolved is we have technology and science. And technology and science have made us aware of the great possibilities in the human potential.

"When Christ lived, his total area of influence was thirty miles. When Buddha lived, his total area of influence was a few hundred miles. Today, with the kind of knowledge that Buddha and Christ gave us, you can go to any bookstore and find 200 books on that subject. And not only is it available, it's available soon through global television. So today we have the ability to bring about a global transformation as it never happened before, and that can only happen if a critical mass of people recognize that pain and suffering is not necessary."

Deepak, as a visionary and healer, is able to provide a unique perspective of our human condition. Through his Center for Well Being, he helps us gain a greater understanding of the true meaning of infinite possibilities. He reminds us of our sacredness and encourages us to contribute our best to the circle of life.

Blase Bonpane, too, recognizes the importance of having a spiritual intention before taking action. Blase is a former Maryknoll priest, community activist, author, teacher, and founder of The Office of the Americas.

Being forcibly disconnected from a community we love is extremely painful, but it can act as a catalyst for showing us our true path in life. Blase shares, "The most disoriented I have ever felt is when I was expelled from Guatemala in 1967. I had established roots with the community, and I loved working and sharing with the people. When I returned to the United States, I felt very much an alien here and I have felt that way ever since."

Blase was catapulted into community activism to make people in the United States aware of what he was witnessing in Guatemala at the time—the political strife, the millions of Guatemalans who were forced into exile, and the North Americans who were ignorant of the plight of these people. Blase felt a rootedness and a connectedness to the people of the community he lived in, and he has been longing for that ever since. He explains, "What they have in their homeland is a community. They have a belongingness that is indescribable. Even money is a matter of the community. If you are about to get married, the community builds your house for you. You don't have to mortgage anything. The worst thing that could happen to you would be to be expelled from the community. When you leave Guatemala, you are no longer categorized as Indian if you change the style of your clothes. If you go to Guatemala City and put on a pair of Levi's and a T-shirt you are technically no longer an Indian. So the matter of being outcast is one of the worst things that can happen to a person."

After Blase returned from Guatemala, he and his wife Teresa continued to do the work that he was doing in the clergy. He shares, "After we had been married for thirteen years our home was no longer inhabitable. It was more of an office—my headquarters for many groups from Latin America or elsewhere. Finally Teresa said, 'We simply have to get this operation out of the house and form a corporation,' which we did. We formed a nonprofit in 1983."

In Blase's experience with re-creating community, he discovered the amazing power of presence. He shares, "You realize that the most important thing we can do in times of trouble is be present to the family that's grieving. During times of political strife, we would simply arrive where a massacre had taken place. The people were so happy to have our presence there to help avoid further massacres of the indigenous people. They could not care less if we were from Scandinavia, Canada, or the United States—because they knew our intentions and could feel what is in our hearts. During crises like Hurricane Mitch we sent money, supplies, and people, and we coordinated it not with just our group, but as a coalition of other concerned communities and organizations. This helped to transform much of our pain and the pain of many others."

We have to come to the understanding about family values and look upon the globe as a family, Blase says. Then we will change our perspectives completely. "Children have to be seen as a privileged class and not as a monetary privileged class. If you have a society that is conscious, children will be the privileged class. We will have the best education for all, the best of services for all, and the best of health care for all. And the people that are the privileged class will be those precisely who are not in a position to take care of their own needs at that time. And we can change this because to make profit the main focus in life, everybody knows is a mistake. People who have worked with money as their only goal are always in pain. They never have enough of it and most people in very, very affluent professions will tell you that. I was speaking to one of the great orthopedic surgeons in the country the other day and he said, 'You know all I was ever interested in was medicine and doing my profession . . . I never even thought about the money. All of a sudden I can't believe it. I have all this money coming in.'

"The main problem we have in the world today is a lack of distributive justice. We have to concentrate on having more distributive justice and never allow words like 'cheap labor' to be used. That's an obscene phrase that violates the human person as a temple of God."

Blase has grown to understand how political activism and spiritual transformation can be very much integrated. He shares, "I see different forms of political action. I think the most effective have been the quasi-religious forms such as the vigil. For example, the other night we did a vigil in our neighborhood where there had been eighteen gang killings. We thought a few people would show up. A thousand people showed up, and we carried candles to each of the sites where people had been shot. We had been told by the police and others that there might be big problems if we did that. Well, that's spiritual transformation and political action together. I have asked in most of the demonstrations for the people to take more of a vigil style approach rather than a screaming, shouting, stomping approach. I see the integration of political activism and spiritual transformation and we see it in Mahatma Gandhi, Nelson Mandela, and Cesar Chavez."

Ela Gandhi is the granddaughter of Mahatma Gandhi, the great world leader for peace and equality. She too understands the necessity of integrating political activism and spiritual transformation. Ela is a member of Parliament, for the African National Congress in South Africa, and is a loved and respected spokesperson for peace and reconciliation.

It is no coincidence that on June 21, 2002, World Peace and Prayer Day was held at the Phoenix settlement in South Africa, the home of the late Mahatma Gandhi. Native American, Indian, African, and people from all walks of life gathered at sunrise on this sacred site to pray for global peace. Chief Arvol Looking Horse, in fulfillment of the Dakota, Lakota, and Nakota prophesies, led the great gathering in prayer. People around the world were also gathered on their sacred sites in prayer, helping to create a worldwide energy shift. After the ceremony, over 8,000 people joined in a march from the Phoenix settlement to the Hindu Temple in Durban.

African traditional healers, African elders, Indian elders, and youth all joined together in a weeklong cultural exchange that renewed old African and Indian connections and created new understanding. There was participation in traditional drumming, gumboots dancing, and Indian dancing. Prayers were offered in many traditions and languages. The gatherings and meals took place at the Temple and other community centers. For the first time since the apartheid rules of separation, thousands of Africans and Indians prayed together in the same temple.

Ela Gandhi hosted the gathering and worked closely with a great team of people from both South Africa and abroad to make this event possible. So heartfelt were the events of that week that Ela's optimism soared. Not since before the terror and devastation by the apartheid regime burning down her grandfather's spiritual community, Phoenix Settlement, and killing hundreds of people in the surrounding community of Inanda, where she grew up, had she felt so much love between the African and Indian people. The apartheid regime's intent was to create separation between the Indian and African population. This was extremely painful for Ela, because she grew up loving and sharing her life with the African people.

Through prayer and applying the principles of forgiveness, peace, and reconciliation, Ela has been able to heal and transform much of her pain. The World Peace and Prayer Day gathering offered a new beginning creating a vision of unity, peace, and reconciliation for Indian and African people.

Mahatma Gandhi's teachings of non-violence have been studied and practiced by millions of people across the globe, including Nelson Mandela and Martin Luther King. For Gandhi, everything started from his resistance against oppression and centered on justice and human rights in a peaceful manner. Ela elaborates, "The beauty in his message is that the whole struggle ends up in reconciliation rather than enmity. Today we look at many forms of oppression and it is common to want to fight oppression with violence, bitterness, and confrontation. But in the end when you have won the battle, there is no reconciliation. So there is no real winner.

"Gandhi fought against oppression, but not against the oppressor.

Today when we see a person or group doing something wrong, we are more likely to destroy that person instead of righting the wrong."

Ela explains that "Gandhi came to South Africa as an ordinary person, a person who was employed by a business to deal with a court case. He came as a middle-class person, who enjoyed living well. But after seeing what the discrimination was doing, that the majority of his own community was accepting discrimination and others were not concerned about it, he began to contemplate and study the writings of great thinkers and leaders. Gandhi's thoughts were guided by people such as Tolstoy and Ruskin and other philosophers. All of these philosophies had an effect on him. He also read the Bhagavad Gita scripture and he went through a major transformation."

Mahatma Gandhi lived the spiritual principles he embraced and inspired people in his own community, as well as diverse communities across the globe, to live a more peaceful and compassionate life with one another. However, today the Phoenix Settlement faces some huge challenges. Ela recounts, "Phoenix Settlement was destroyed on a Friday, and on Sunday, two days later, truckloads of people arrived and people were just dumped there. I don't know who brought them. But they were brought and told that they could build their homes on the land. People were given materials and pieces of land and within a few days there were hundreds of shacks on the Phoenix Settlement. And then more people turned up and there were fights against them and they went and burned down the whole settlement. Hundreds of shacks were burned down, and hundreds of people were killed on the settlement. Today we have a kind of double battle. On the one hand trying to help people to understand what the Phoenix Settlement is all about and why it's necessary for people to respect the place and the land. The other great concern is to help the people to develop themselves. People used to call the settlement, 'The place of God.' It was respected like one would respect a church. But those were the old days and those were the old people. We knew what the settlement stood for and we respected it. That is the kind of environment we grew up in."

As part of the World Peace and Prayer Day delegation, my daughter and I witnessed the healing efforts taking place among the people of the community. I returned home remembering that Africa is referred to as the cradle of humanity, and with the realization that there in South Africa people are choosing paths of healing, reconciliation, and peace.

Ela works with wonderful and dedicated people who were committed to World Peace and Prayer Day and who represent the Indian and African communities. Two gentlemen who have moved me deeply are Lenford Moibi and Seelan Achary. They both are leaders of their respective African and Indian communities, and have joined forces not only to carry forth the event but even more profoundly to renew healthy relations between the African and Indian people. Both Seelan and Lenford along with others have committed themselves wholeheartedly to the transformation of Bhambayi and the surrounding community of Inanda. Both African and Indian people are coming together to listen to their elders talk about what really happened during the violence that has created such heartache and loss in the community. In the spirit of Ubuntu and the principles of non-

violence and self-sufficiency that Gandhi embraced, they are coura-
geously and lovingly re-creating their community.

Clearly it will take time for many of the people of South Africa to
wipe out the colonial legacy. The struggle continues as they move
towards the emergence of a society that will enable their children
and the future generations to lead secure, comfortable, and happy
lives. The universal truths of peace and reconciliation speak to us all.

All of these stories reveal that every individual can have an impact
in making our local communities as well as global community more
loving and peaceful. Community can be in the form of a town, or it
can be spiritual, or it can be a manifestation of our values and interests. Ultimately it is about being connected to another and recognizing and celebrating that realization in each other. On our individual
healing journeys, there is much that connects us. When we live in
alignment with universal truths and laws, we are able to live a balanced and harmonious life with all of natural creation. We discover
our place in the circle of life and are able to live in accordance with
our true nature. We understand that the oasis of well-being resides
within our heart, and in reaching out to one another we create a joyous oneness.

Conclusion

Writing this book has taken both me and my daughter on a life-changing journey. I have learned a most important lesson—that when you give of yourself, you are blessed and provided for in more ways than you can imagine. I also learned to stay connected to the life force that makes all things possible, and to listen to my inner guidance. It became more and more clear to me to trust the Divine for my source and supply. I learned to create my path and stay in alignment with universal principles. And finally, through this journey, I have found my voice, for so long wavering and tentative. I have learned how to become stronger in who I am and what I am here to do.

The truth that we are connected with everyone and everything became especially clear as I was entrusted with the precious life stories, experiences, and perceptions of extraordinary healers, visionaries, creative artists, and peacemakers in this book. Although I did not see them on a daily basis, I felt more and more connected to them because I was carrying their words and essence in my heart. I felt as if they were a part of me and I a part of them. It was surprising how each time I was re-editing and writing, I would discover an important message in a story that I was not ready or able to hear before. There was a constant unfolding, a reminder of how in life, things also unfold and reveal themselves.

A common theme running through people's lives is the realization that forgiveness is a key to a happier life. On this journey, I was guided to a book called *Radical Forgiveness* by Colin Tipping. I was still somewhat stuck with feeling "victimized" by a circumstance in my life, and I was unable to really free myself of that feeling. The book literally fell off the bookshelf onto the floor in front of me. The first page I turned to showed me that the harsh circumstance that I was experiencing was a valuable life lesson. My entire perspective shifted. *Radical Forgiveness* assists us in undoing what has caused pain in our lives. It acts on our psyche in such a way as to enable us to let go of the victim archetype, open our hearts, and raise our vibration. I was ready to do some real forgiveness work. My life took a major turn from that moment. For me the gift of pain has been to greatly expand my awareness of unity with everyone and everything. It has led me to understand the power of forgiveness to bring greater peace and joy into my life.

So many people have great concern about the need for peace and reconciliation on Earth. And I have grown to understand that world peace is connected to each person's inner peace. I realized that the inner work that I needed to do was a perfect continuation of the awareness that I gained in the favelas of Brazil, the Native American reservations, the inner city of Los Angeles, and the communities in South Africa.

Having recently returned from South Africa as part of the World Peace and Prayer Day delegation hosted by Ela Gandhi and led by Chief Arvol Looking Horse, I was both humbled and inspired by the realization that we truly can create an energy shift on Mother Earth, one that reminds us that we are all connected and we are all sacred. Our pain has brought us to this realization. Now it is time to understand the gift of our experiences and together focus on caring for one another and all of natural creation.

Contributor Contact Information

Isabel Allende
www.isabelallende.com

Butch Artichoker
Fax: (605)856-5390
bwing@gwtc.net

Margaret Ayers
(310)276-9181
www.neuropathways.com

Reverend Michael Beckwith
Agape International Spiritual Center
5700 Buckingham Parkway
Culver City, CA 90230
(310)348-1250
www.agapelive.com

Blase Bonpane
Office of the Americas
8124 West Third St., Suite 202
Los Angeles, CA 90048
(323)852-0808

Joan Borysenko
Mind/Body Health Sciences
393 Bixon Rd.
Boulder, CO 80302
(303)440-8460
Fax: (303)440-7530
www.joanborysenko.com

Barbara Brennan
500 NW Spanish River, Suite 10B
Boca Raton, FL 33431-4559
(561)338-9155
Fax: (561)338-4776
www.barbarabrennan.com

Rickie Byars-Beckwith
rickiebb@agapelive.com

Jack Canfield
www.jackcanfield.com
www.chickensoup.com

Deepak Chopra
Chopra Center at La Costa Resort and Spa
7321 Estrella De Mar Rd.
Carlsbad, CA 92009
(888)424-6722
www.chopra.com

Bernie Dohrmann
www.IBIGlobal.com

Dr. Larry Dossey, M.D.
Executive Editor

Alternative Therapies
878 Paseo Del Sur
Santa Fe, NM 87501
(505)986-8188
Fax: (505)986-1614
www.dosseydossey.com

Linda Fickes
Fickes Holistic Care Corp.
4224 Wailae Ave., Suite 5-335
Honolulu, HI 96816
(808)377-1811
drfickes@hawaii.rr.com
www.lovelife.com/breastthermography

Lenny Foster
Len.Foster@nndoh.org

John Funmaker
Sundance Family Wellness Center
1614 W. Temple
Los Angeles, CA 90026
(213)353-9429

Ela Gandhi
egandhi@anc.org.za

Dick Gregory
www.dickgregory.com

Alaine Haubert
al.haubert@verizon.net

William Herskovic
freedmanfilms@aol.com

Gerry Jampolsky and Diane Cirincione
Center for Attitudinal Healing
33 Buchanan Dr.
Sausalito, CA 94965
(415)331-6161
Fax: (415)331-4545
http://attitudinalhealing.org

Dr. Ibrahim Karim
International Institute for Bau-Biologic and Ecology, Inc.
P.O. Box 387
Clearwater, FL 33757
baubiologie@earthlink.net
www.bau-biologieusa.com

Steven Lewis
(310)656-7828
www.energeticmatrix.com

Chief Arvol Looking Horse
www.wolakota.org
www.worldpeaceandprayerday.org

Miriam Lynette
P.O. Box 32722
Santa Fe, NM 87594
Fax: (505)474-4524

Rigoberta Menchú Tum
Heriberto Frias 339
Col. Navarte
03020 Mexico D.F. Mexico
Phone/Fax: (52)5639-3091-5639-1492

frmtmexico@rigobertamenchu.org
www.rigobertamenchu.org

Auntie Momie (Marie Leimomi)
219 Crest Ave.
Wahiawa, HI 96786
(808)622-4747

Afrika Msimang
Tswelopele Renaissance School
P.O. Box 421
Kelvin 2054, Gauteng, South Africa
Afrika06@yahoo.com

Dr. Roy Nakai
125 W. Franklin St.
Lake Elsinore, CA 93530
(949)439-0596
fforrester@mindspring.com

Kahu O Te Range
akulele@aol.com

Rabbi Zalman Schachter-Shalomi
www.spiritualeldering.org
www.aleph.org

Jana Shiloh
life@sedona.net

Iyanla Vanzant
(301)608-8750
www.innervisionsworldwide.com

Dr. Tobin Watkinson
Scripps Health Medical Offices
12395 El Camino Real, Suite 300
San Diego, CA 92130
(858)793-0211
DRTOBYW@aol.com

Dr. Tobin Watkinson
Scripps Health Medical Offices
12395 El Camino Real, Suite 300
San Diego, CA 92130
(858)793-0211
DRTOBYW@aol.com

Energy Medicine Resources

Books Explaining Energy Medicine

The Energy Within, Richard M. Chin, M.D., O.M.D.

Vibrational Medicine, Richard Gerber, M.D.

Sources of Energy Medicine

Homeopathic *Arnica* is in health-food stores, and we use it before and after surgery and injury.

Flower remedies are in health-food stores, and Dr. Bach's *Rescue Remedy* is widely used for shock, emotional stress, headaches, and much more.

Energems are small, attractive energized mineral transmitters that neutralize environmental toxins such as electromagnetic, geopathic, and atmospheric stresses. Toll-free (866)815-0696; *www.energems.com*.

Vital Force Energetic Formulas are precisely targeted to have a profound effect on energy reserves and overall health, whether physiological or psychological. (800)341-7458; *www.energytoolsint.com*.

Sound Wave Energy uses sound frequences in CD forms to create harmony and balance at the physical, emotional, mental, and spiritual levels. (888)267-2309; *www.harmonyera.com*.

Index